COLON CANCER
PATIENT ADVOCATE

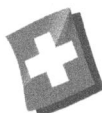

HealthScouter
WWW.HEALTHSCOUTER.COM

HealthScouter.com - Equity Press
5055 Canyon Crest Drive
Riverside, California 92507

www.healthscouter.com

Purchasing this book entitles you to free updates at www.healthscouter.com/colon_cancer

Edited By: Kathy Wong

Includes Colon Cancer from Wikipedia http://en.wikipedia.org/wiki/colon_cancer

HealthScouter Colon Cancer: Colon Cancer Symptoms, Colon Cancer Early Symptoms (HealthScouter Colon Cancer)

ISBN 978-1-60332-072-6

Important

NEVER DISREGARD PROFESSIONAL MEDICAL ADVICE, OR DELAY SEEKING IT, BECAUSE OF SOMETHING YOU HAVE READ IN THIS BOOK. ALWAYS SEEK PROFESSIONAL MEDICAL ADVICE BEFORE ACTING UPON INFORMATION READ IN THIS BOOK.

HealthScouter and Equity Press do not provide medical advice. The contents of this book are for informational purposes only and are not intended to substitute for professional medical advice, diagnosis or treatment. Always seek advice from a qualified physician or health care professional about any medical concern, and do not disregard professional medical advice because of anything you may read in this book or on a HealthScouter Web site. The views of individuals quoted in this book are not necessarily those of HealthScouter or Equity Press.

While this book is intended to be a medium for the exchange of information and ideas, it is not meant in any way to be a substitute for sound medical advice; neither should it be viewed as a trusted source of such advice. The views expressed in these messages are not those of any qualified medical association, and the publisher is not responsible for the validity of the information communicated herein or for consequences that may arise from acting upon this information. The publisher is not responsible for any content found in the book that may be deemed offensive, inappropriate, inaccurate or medically unsound. The information you find here is only for the purpose of discussion and should not be the basis for any medical decision. The content is not intended to be a substitute for professional medical advice, diagnosis or treatment.

The information presented is not to be considered complete, nor does it contain all medical resource information that may be relevant, and therefore it is not intended to be a substitute for seeking medical treatment and/or appropriate care.

By reading this book and parts of the Web site, you agree under all circumstances to hold harmless, and to refrain from seeking remedy from, the owners of this book. The publisher shall disclaim all liability to you for damages, costs or expenses, including legal and medical fees, related to your reliance on anything derived from this book or Web site or its contents. Furthermore, Equity Press assumes no liability for any and all claims arising out of the said use, regardless of the cause, effects, or fault.

Equity Press and HealthScouter do not endorse any company or product, and listing on the HealthScouter Web site is not linked to corporate sponsorship. We do not make a claim to being comprehensive or up to date. If you would like to recommend information to include in this book, please contact us – we would be very happy to hear from you.

Purchasing this book entitles you to free updates as they are available. Please register your book at www.healthscouter.com

TABLE OF CONTENTS

INTRODUCTION AND MOTIVATION

Dear Reader,

I like to think of myself as a polite, well-reasoned person. I rarely speak out or complain. When a waitress spills something on me, or if my meal is cold—or if I'm overcharged—I generally try to be as polite as possible. I don't like to make very many waves. I often secretly hope that the manager will hear about my predicament and come out and offer me a free meal, or something similar. I generally hope that my polite and respectful demeanor pays off. And it does happen from time to time. You know, I think many people are brought up to believe that this is just good manners. It's how you're supposed to behave. And if you knew me personally, I think you'd agree that I'm generally pretty reserved. Of course my wife may raise an objection or two (!), but I really believe that it's important to treat others as you would like to be treated. We're talking about the golden rule here—it works well and it applies to almost every life circumstance.

But I have to admit that when it comes to my health, or the health of someone I care about—all bets are off. I want to know what's going on—when, why, where, and how. And I make these feelings known. I tend to get downright assertive. It's just something I feel very strongly about. And I feel that when you are in a hospital, or if you're brushing up against the healthcare system, that you should feel the same way. It's unfamiliar turf, and the professionals who work in this system often take advantage of their positions. They may use some jargon to hide the whole truth— or they may say something without checking to make sure you understand completely. They may present the options that are best for them, perhaps the most profitable or convenient. Now I'm not saying this goes on everywhere. There are many professionals in the business of health who go out of their way to make sure you have the best care. And I'm not suggesting that you should become a bully, or purposefully annoying—absolutely not. But I am suggesting that I think it's OK for you to step outside of your typical comfort zone, and put on your patient advocate hat. Because you, the patient or patient advocate, care the most about your care—not the medical system or healthcare providers.

HealthScouter was created to help patients become better advocates for their own medical care. Because when it comes to your healthcare, the stakes are high. There are none higher. And healthcare is one area where consumers (us, the sick people) are notoriously unaware of their options. And that's why I'm publishing these books. To help you understand your options, and to help you get the best care possible. I want to help you become a better advocate for yourself and for your loved ones.

It's my sincere hope that you can take this book with you to the hospital, to be read in the waiting room or by the bedside—and when you see a relevant patient comment you can use this book to ask questions of your health care providers. My advice: Ask lots of questions! Providers are busy people who generally go about their business with little questioning, delivering care as they see fit—making quick decisions—and again, nobody is going to care as much about your health as you. So now, more than ever, you need tools at your disposal to get the best care possible. One of the tools at your disposal is this HealthScouter book and the material within. You need to be armed with questions, and you need to ask questions all of the time. And so the difficult part is now to understand the right questions to ask.

That brings me to an explanation of how these books are structured. HealthScouter books include a number of what we call patient comments. These patient comments are summaries of what people have experienced. They're first hand accounts of what you may expect. These experiences effectively help you "catch up," and understand what outcomes are possible. They expose you to the treatments are available, and provide insight as to potential outcomes. They help you understand what other people are doing. So if you find yourself stuck feeling like you're receiving substandard medical care—or if you need a push to broach the subject, you can take this book to your provider and say, "Hey, I read here that another patient had this treatment—is that an option for me? If not, Why?" I believe that other peoples' experience is the most valuable way for you to formulate and build a list of good questions for your healthcare providers.

That notion is at the core of the HealthScouter philosophy.

So HealthScouter, by providing patient comments about a particular medical condition, will help expose you to what other people have experienced about a particular medical problem. If you know what other people have experienced, you can better understand what your options are. You'll be better informed and you'll have some questions to ask—it'll be like you've had access to dozens of other people who have gone through the same thing you're going through. And so armed, maybe you'll be able to move through your condition and get back on the road to health, and maybe you'll be able to do this with more grace than I have. And that is my sincere wish.

It's also my wish that perhaps when a doctor or nurse sees this little blue book, that they'll think twice about the care they're about to provide—knowing that the owner is a little bit better prepared, a little bit better armed—and yes, maybe even downright assertive.

I hope this book helps.

Yours truly,

Jim Stewart

San Diego, California

HOW TO USE THIS BOOK

The purpose of HealthScouter is to help you understand your medical condition as quickly and easily as possible. We believe this can best be accomplished by reading about other people and their experiences negotiating their health and care. We try to leave out complicated medical jargon. And we've spent a considerable amount of time structuring this book so that it's easy to use. It's important to know that this is not the sort of book you read from beginning to end. Of course you may do so, but this book is more meaningful if you flip through quickly and scan for applicable material. Again, it's all about the patient commentary: The darkly shaded comments � indicate one patient initiating a new discussion, and the light or clear comments ⌑ are other comments associated with that same condition. So you should begin by looking for information from other patients who are experiencing the same aspect of the same medical condition that you studying. You can do this quickly by scanning through the book, focusing on the dark shaded comment boxes. By scanning the patient comments you'll find information about various aspects of a condition, all grouped together, in an easy-to-read format. In this way you can immediately begin reading about other patients and their experiences with your particular medical condition – and you can benefit immediately from their experiences.

COLORECTAL CANCER

From Wikipedia, the free encyclopedia

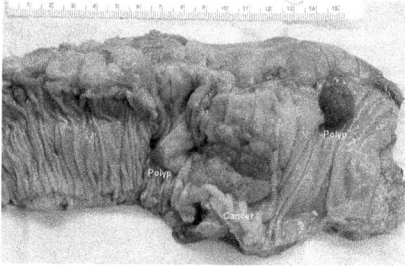

Gross appearance of a colectomy specimen containing two adenomatous polyps (the dark oval tumors above the labels, attached to the normal lining by a stalk) and one invasive colorectal carcinoma (the crater-like, irregularly-shaped tumor located above the label).

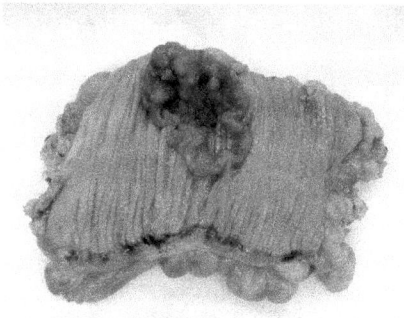

Gross appearance of a colectomy specimen containing one invasive colorectal carcinoma (the crater-like, irregularly-shaped tumor).

Colorectal cancer, also called colon cancer or large bowel cancer, includes cancerous growths in the colon, rectum and appendix. With 655,000 deaths worldwide per year, it is the third most common form of cancer and the second leading cause of cancer-related death in the Western world.[1] Many colorectal cancers are thought to arise from adenomatous polyps in the colon. These mushroom-like growths are usually benign, but some may develop into cancer over time. The majority of the time, the diagnosis of localized colon cancer is through colonoscopy. Therapy is usually through surgery, which in many cases is followed by chemotherapy.

I'm 20, and a little over a week ago I had a bowel movement that came out really flat and ribbony. About a week ago, when I had a bowel movement, it was slightly thicker than it was, but still nowhere close to normal. A few days ago my bowel movement is still getting slightly better but it's still really ribbony. The last couple days, the bowel movement was normal. But when I took a bowel movement again yesterday, it was ribbony again. Then today, it was still ribbony. It has been a normal color. I wonder if stress, diet, or exercising less than normal can cause weird bowel movements like this. Abdominal distension: Nope. Abdominal pain: Nope. Unexplained, persistent nausea

or vomiting: Nope. Unexplained weight loss: Nope. Change in frequency or character of stool (bowel movements): Yep. Small-caliber (narrow) or ribbon-like stools: Yep. Sensation of incomplete evacuation after a bowel movement: Nope. Rectal pain: Nope. Age. About 90 percent of people diagnosed with colon cancer are older than 50; I'm 20. A personal history of colorectal cancer or polyps: Not that I know of. Inflammatory intestinal conditions: Nope. Inherited disorders that affect the colon: I might have hemorrhoids, though it usually doesn't cause a problem for me. Basically it's not active most of the time. Family history of colon cancer and colon polyps: Only my grandma, nobody else even polyps. Diet: Colon cancer and rectal cancer may be associated with a diet low in fiber and high in fat and calories: Probably. A sedentary lifestyle: Yes, but I do try to get at least a little bit of exercise each day. Diabetes: Nope. Obesity: I'm only 129 pounds. Smoking: a smoker. I really hope it's just my obsessive/ compulsive disorder doing this to me. Sadly, my parents would just get mad at me for wanting to go to the doctors for this. I've sort of been worrying about so many things that they just think that I'm just worrying too much again, though they have been right every time they've told me not to worry.

I am pretty sure that though it is more common for someone in their fifties to get colon cancer, someone in their twenties or thirties can get it as well. It is rare but it has happened.

I have read that there does not have to be blood in the stool as a cancer indicator. Ribboned stools can be a sign of colon cancer but do not automatically mean that a person has colon cancer. I think the best thing for a person who is experiencing these signs and symptoms is to go to a specialist and have a battery of tests done to rule out cancer and any other bowel diseases.

Colon cancer could be from stress and worry, but I think confirming this with a doctor is the best and smartest thing to do. I will do it for myself because my health comes first and I am the only one who can do something about it.

I just got the horrible news that I have rectal cancer. I'm only 56. The worst information was that the tumor is so close to the muscle that I will most likely have to have a colostomy. I begin six weeks of chemo and radiation next week and then will have surgery sometime eight to ten weeks later. I've decided to let the surgeons do a total hysterectomy at the same time so it can't come back there. I have been having a colonoscopy every three years for the last nine years. They have removed little polyps each time I've gone in and all in the past had been fine. This tumor wasn't there the last time, so I can't begin to stress the importance in getting checked. I was due for my three-year recheck and noticed bright red blood on the outside of the stool and had thought that it might be an internal hemorrhoid. My PET/CT scan showed that it has moved to other organs, yet they gave me a number of T2 for depth of the tumor. We still don't know if the lymph nodes are involved and won't know for sure until the surgery. If they are, then I begin chemo again after the surgery. I know I have a great team of doctors, but if I don't become educated, I won't really know what to ask them.

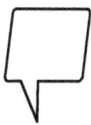

I believe that there is a cure for cancer, and it's not found in conventional medicine. I know people trust their doctors now, and I do hope everyone will be cancer-free. Anyway, if anything goes wrong with the "treatments" doctors offer, one shouldn't lose hope or give up. That is the time for people to go alternative. There are, for example, treatments with iodine, sodium bicarbonate, etc. I know this can sound outrageous to many doctors, but I also know how much cancer patients need real help/cure when conventional medicine fails.

I was diagnosed with ST3 colon CA at age 48. It was very aggressive and into six lymph nodes. I had surgery and a year of chemo. Next month will be the start of year 12 CA free.

My husband was diagnosed over five years ago with ST 111C and is doing well today. He was told he would need a colostomy but they managed to avoid that. The only side effect he has is urgency.

There are people who live normal lives with colostomies; I shouldn't be too disheartened if I have to have one. Of course, it is scary but I believe I could adjust. I am sure someone will encourage me with that.

I was one month shy of my fiftieth birthday when I was diagnosed with ST 3 rectal cancer. After six weeks of chemo and radiation, I had pouch surgery. This surgery was to not only remove the rectum, but also to save the sphincter muscle. I did have to have an ileostomy until the colon healed from the surgery. I then had six more months of chemo. After the loop closure, the ileostomy was removed and I now use my new "rectum." I have some issues with urgency and diarrhea, but better than a permanent ileostomy pouch. I would suggest anyone with a diagnosis similar to mine seek out a surgeon who specializes in colon cancer. The first surgeon I met with was a general surgeon who told me I would probably lose my sphincter muscles and have a permanent ostomy pouch. Not so when speaking with the colon specialist. I must find a surgeon who knows the J pouch procedure. I have been working for two years to get to this point, and my new normal is allowing me to live a full life.

The surgeon I met with is a specialist in colo/rectal surgery, and he said because of the location of the tumor (approx 1 cm. away from the sphincter), it just wasn't enough room to be able to remove the tumor and attach the tissue and save the sphincter. He said it would come back if he doesn't give a buffer of room.

I love my oncologist and the radiologist—they are truly very special caring people, but one surgeon was just plain insensitive, almost to the point of *being rude when he gave me the news. I will probably seek a second opinion at some point while I'm going through chemo and radiation. Everyone says that the surgeon is very gifted as it pertains to his specialty, but he should never be allowed to talk to a patient. At the very least, he could have said that as he was doing the surgery, he would try and do everything possible to excise the tumor without damaging the sphincter.*

I was on emotional overload while researching colon cancer and the J pouch. I just can't seem to stop crying, and I know I need to get to a point where I'm mad so I can start figuring out what to do.

My husband and I have the same oncologist, as we both have/had cancer and I love him dearly. As to the surgeon, some have a way of saying the most upsetting things. Can you imagine when I got my diagnosis of lymphoma, one said to me, "Will it kill you? Well, possibly but probably not for some years yet." Luckily, he was not the one who first gave me the diagnosis.

Anyone with colon cancer may have to weigh up the fact that their surgeon is so well skilled in his specialty versus a total lack of bedside manner. I discovered that too much research could overload me. It can be so overwhelming.

People can find the strength to fight cancer. I really like this quote: "Anyone can give up; it's the easiest thing in the world to do. But to hold it together when everyone else would understand if you fell apart, that's true strength."

With regard to colon cancer surgery, I advise exploring the possibility of having the J pouch procedure and finding a great surgeon. My tumor was so low in the rectum, the doctor could feel the tumor through physical exam. That is how low my tumor was and how close it was to the sphincter. I also didn't look for a specialist until I got my head together. This was during radiation and my first round of chemo. I would suggest that patients look as soon as possible, before the treatments cause weakness. As far as the ostomy goes, I hated it. But, it would have been fine if I had to have had it forever. A person can adjust, and if it is choosing between an ostomy and my family, no contest! I focus on my inner peace and find my blessings, then trudge forward.

I was diagnosed almost six years ago with rectal cancer. I had a temporary ileo for six months with hopes my colon would heal and it would be reversed. Unfortunately due to previous issues, my colon did not heal and I decided to have the ileo changed to a permanent colostomy. After a few months of learning to adjust, I know that a colostomy does not slow me down. I have always been very active and continue to travel—golfing, scuba diving, hiking, biking, running, swimming, cross country skiing, and weight training as easily as before. I also wear exactly the same style of clothing as before. The more I learned about treatments and surgery, the easier it for me and I felt more confident and positive about the outcome. If a colostomy is recommended for anyone, I highly recommend seeing an ET (stoma/wound) nurse for information before surgery.

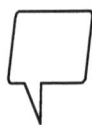

I might have to have a colostomy. I've heard that it is possible to wear the same clothes. But I don't understand how it won't it show through. How does a person go swimming? We cruise a lot and sometimes lay by the pool. I'm afraid I have to be in one of those granny-type suits. I've seen some stuff on the Web that scared the heck out of me and now I'm confused. One video had someone giving a demo on a big plastic thing that looked like a garbage bag girdle with a vacuum pump on it. I just about lost it on that one.

My husband had his colonoscopy today and all was fine. While I was there, I spoke with his doctor. She gave me the name of a couple of colo/rectal surgeons who she says might either give me some hope or at worst confirm what the other doctor said.

My stoma sits below and to the left of my belly button. I have an incision that starts slightly below my belly button but is not very obvious. I wear a regular two-piece suit that is a "hipster" style. We can get ostomy appliances that are so thin, soft, and flexible that when empty no one would ever know anything is there. It is important that if anyone requires a colostomy to have the stoma placed low enough if possible to still wear "non-granny" jeans, etc. I do know of some people in my support group that seem to go out of the way to wear the most baggy and unattractive clothes, as if it is now required. Totally wrong! But then at my age I probably shouldn't be wearing two-piece swimsuits, but I do anyway. There's a very famous climber by the name of Rob Hill who started a group called "No Guts Know Glory" who is climbing the world's tallest mountains. He has an ileostomy—a real inspiration!

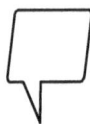

I just spoke with my oncologist regarding the names of the additional colo/rectal surgeons I obtained yesterday. I wanted to see if he knew of them. Although he says it's fine to get a second opinion, there is no hope that they can spare me from a colostomy since the sphincter muscle is basically involved and, even if the tumor shrinks, there isn't a chance that they can save the muscle. I'll try and find a support group since I know I need to move forward.

I was diagnosed with rectal cancer four years ago and chose to have no treatment after the mass was removed, but to aggressively monitor with CEA and CT scans every three months. I thought I was doing great until this week. My CEA jumped from 3.6 to 7.9 in less than three months. I am still a smoker and my doctor has been monitoring a 6 mm. nodule (uncalcified) for change. It's been over a year and it does not show any changes, yet the CEA has freaked me out. I suppose it has also freaked out my doctor because he sent me to a surgeon and I am having a PET done. The surgeon said that it will be a "challenge" to do the surgery, due to *its "deep, centered" location, and I will have to have the VATS surgery even though at 6 mm., it might not show up on a PET. Due to the location of the nodule, he might not be able to do it laproscopically. I am now also scheduled for yet another CT next week. I haven't stopped crying long enough to look up any information, but he did say that the pain would be "considerable." I am terrified.*

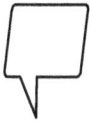

At the age of 43, I had a nodule in my right upper lobe. They did CT scans every three months and on the sixth month it tripled in size and became "speculated." The PET scan showed "hypermedobolic uptake," which can indicate cancer. I was scheduled for a staging procedure called EBUS/EUS with biopsies of the lymph nodes as well as a brushing and washing of the mass, which were inconclusive. I was scheduled for an open thoracotomy and a right upper lobectomy. By the grace of God it wasn't cancer! It was negative for TB, fungal, pneumonia, viral, etc. It took several weeks for the diagnosis, which turned out to be a rare infection called MAC or MAI (mycobacterial avium-intracellular complex). There is an upswing with this infection, particularly in middle-aged women, and the National Institute

of Health, National Jewish, as well as University of Texas have all been doing major research with this infection. It's been around a long time and originally was associated with HIV-AIDS, but now this upswing is linked to young women that do not have HIV or AIDS, and it is confined within the lungs, unlike people who are HIV positive where it is throughout their bodies but not in their lungs. They are searching for a common gene marker for why women are getting this infection. My biggest surprise was that many doctors are not updated about this infection or never even heard of it, and those who have heard of it still associate it with HIV. It's scary for sure just finding a doctor that has the knowledge to treat this. Anyway, my point is that my MAC did not present typical. It presented like cancer in a solitary spiculated nodule. Usually there are multiple nodules with MAC, so it is possible to have MAC with only one nodule.

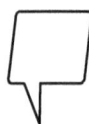

I had my surgery in November of last year, and I now have two micronodules in my right lung and another in my left lung. I've opted to wait and see and do a high resolution CT scan in February and see what is going on in there. This infection can be very difficult to treat, and at this point I'm in that zone where they don't know for sure if this is MAC as well or something new brewing. So we will see. My pulmonologist has told me that if I have anything new to come in right away for testing. So I do feel like he is looking in my best interest.

With regard to pain from colorectal surgery, being firm with one's doctor as to what can be taken for pain is vital. One should look up information on pain meds as well. Some doctors are scared to give anything more than a Tylenol. I have even had doctors tell me they had to fight for pain meds for their relatives. My grandson had cancer surgery and upfront told the surgeon what he was deathly allergic to and what would work and only to give him that or he wasn't doing the surgery. The doctor listened. Even for tests, I now know to tell the doctors what I am going to do to relieve my anxiety and pain or I am not doing it. When I explained my position to the lung doctor, he wrote out the prescriptions and said just tell the hospital what I had taken before arriving. It makes the tests a lot easier to do.

I went for a year playing the guessing game, which did more on my nerves and left me little time to enjoy life. A person can't heal without knowing what one is dealing with.

It might be a good idea to get copies of one's surgery report, CT scan reports, doctor reports, as well as lab and culture results to have accurate information to share with other medical providers as well as to help understand what was done and found.

I have a 3 cm. rectal polyp and it bleeds sometimes but there is no pain. I am 35 years old and am terrified to death.

Usually with polyps, or at that point benign tumors, they are removed by colon resection if they cannot be removed (when they are smaller) during colonoscopy. I have never heard of them being left. I had a similar problem where two tumors were in my right side colon. I had a right hemi-colectomy in 2006 to remove them and to further test for cancer. They came back benign, but I have a colonoscopy every year to cut out the new growths which are always there. I have grown anywhere from three to six in a year.

Eight years ago, my father was diagnosed with rectal cancer (stage T4N1). After surviving surgery/chemo/radiation therapy, he lived a normal life until one-and-a-half yeas ago when his CEA level began to rise. PET scan

revealed two hyper-metabolic spots in his
thoracic spine, suggesting bony metastasis.
He was otherwise asymptomatic except that
his renal function is on the low side (serum
creatinin ~130–150). Subsequently, he was put
on FOLFOX (Capecitabine [Xeloda], Oxaliplatin
[Eloxatin]) in combination with Avastin. My
father at age ~70 responded well to the drug
regime as his CEA dropped from ~90 (before
chemo) to ~5 (near end of chemo). Then, his
CEA was on the rise again, up to 68. CT scan
showed no abnormality in major organs. At that
point, he started undergoing another course
of chemo with infusional 5-fluorouracil and
irinotecan (CPT-11). After finishing his 5th cycle
out of 10, he was taken off from the treatment
as his CEA rises further to ~130. Apparently,
he is not responding to CPT-11 at all. Now we
are considering yet another course of chemo
involving Cetuximab [Erbitux], radiation therapy
or CyberKnife radiosurgery as a preventive
measure to treat his bony metastasis problem,
or no further aggressive treatment. Given what
he has gone through recently, we fear that
he may not respond favorably to yet another
chemo drug combination. We're wondering if it
would be useful to go back to a previously-tried

chemo drug (e.g., Xeloda). In light of his overall CEA trend, we are curious about how soon any symptoms (due to metastasis) will begin to surface.

It is hard to estimate what symptoms might appear with rectal cancer, or when they will arise. I don't think even a doctor could pinpoint that. It could be days to months.

Somewhere I read of a person's CEA going up in the 800s. There are sites that have copies of articles on CEA from medical journals. Just recently I was reading about the numbers being related to the "volume of the tumor," whatever that means (perhaps size of the mass). I don't know. In the past when mine goes up to 2.5, I get sent for a CT scan. The last one was 2.8, and I'm scheduled for a PET.

I was diagnosed in June of 2005 with stage IIIC rectal cancer. It was a very aggressive cancer. I had a hysterectomy and lower resection. I had two weeks of chemo treatment and then a month of chemo and radiation together. I had many problems during the treatments. I was allergic to 5FU and ended up in the hospital for two weeks because of lowered white blood cells. I am three years after treatment, with no cancer, *but many medical issues. I have severe lower back pain, bone pain, fatigue, chemo brain, nausea, cramping, and four to six urgent bowel movements a day. I thought it would get better. I cannot stand longer than 45 minutes without severe pain. If I overdo it, I run a fever and end up in bed for two days sick and with lower back pain.*

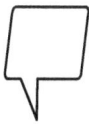

I found that vitamin D works well for bone pain. Maybe people with bone pain should get their vitamin D levels checked.

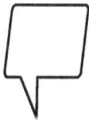

I was diagnosed in 1998 with aggressive Stage 3 colon cancer into 6 lymph glands. It was removed and I had 48 weekly sessions of 5FU enhanced with levamisole. Since then I have had no sign of cancer, but I have had pancreatis, had my gallbladder removed, passed several kidney stones, had elevated cholesterol, and am borderline diabetic with insulin resistance. I was recently diagnosed with a serious kidney disease called minimal change disease that has been unsuccessfully treated with long-term, high dose prednisone. My doctor now suspects that it is a more serious condition called which nearly always ends in renal failure. It has been nearly eleven

years of survival, but my quality of life has been very poor.

My mother was recently diagnosed with Stage 4 colon cancer, which has spread to other areas around her colon. They cannot remove the main tumor because it is too big, so the plan is to shrink it first then hopefully go back in and remove it. The oncologist has her starting chemo, but not radiation. My understanding is chemo has a chance to shrink it, but why not try both at the same time? I understand the radiation will not do anything for the other cancer in her liver and the surrounding areas, but why not give her chemo for that, and also use radiation directed at the big tumor? I asked the oncologist but they didn't really explain it too well.

My understanding is that radiation therapy is not a common way to treat colon cancer, though it may be used in certain circumstances—not sure why.

I also was diagnosed with Stage 4 colorectal cancer which had spread to my liver. My team of oncologists and surgeons had me undergo chemo 5FU for five weeks as well as radiation that was directed at the colon tumor. We allowed six weeks for the tumors to shrink, and then I had surgery to remove two-thirds of my liver and 12 inches of colon. That was two weeks ago and as of today I am cancer free. I will begin six months of chemo to help ensure that the cancer does not return. From the research I have done, my experience is typical for treatment of colorectal cancer which has spread.

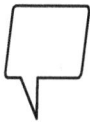

I had Stage 3 rectal cancer and had to have two weeks of chemo, then one month of radiation and chemo together. It was difficult and a long journey toward healing. One can only heal with family and friends and God to help. Good doctors that one can trust make all the difference in the world. It's a must to form a team of doctors that will work with and give one all the info needed. I go to the library and bookstore and read all the books I can about rectal cancer. Colon cancer is a little different than rectal cancer—different treatment and side effects.

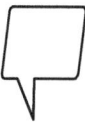

Expectations vary depending on health at time of diagnosis, state of primary tumors, and how secondaries are developing. Here is my husband's timeline of events:

- April 2003 (aged 44) diagnosed at Stage 4 with multiple mets to liver. He had lost about 30 percent of his body weight.

- May 2003 low anterior resection, no bag.
- June–August 2003 6 cycles of Oxaliplatin/5fu/ leucrovin (this reduced sizes of liver tumors to operable level).
- September 2003 liver resection.
- December 2003 one month of daily radiotherapy with continuous 5fu.
- March–May 2004 final 6 cycles of Oxaliplatin/ 5fu/leucrovin; the final 6 cycles were considered to offer protection against recurrence although at that time there was not a lot of evidence to support this.

He has been clear since his treatment stopped. At his last checkup with liver surgeon this year, they decided to keep him on the books and not discharge him, as there is now growing evidence that a very small number of Oxaliplatin users are showing recurrence. They just want to keep checking him for a few more years beyond the five-year threshold. We consider ourselves lucky that he is still around at all, as his prognosis at diagnosis was extremely poor.

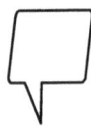

My husband's doctor acknowledged that his pain is real. He ordered another CT scan and PET scan and then a bone scan (first one). The doctor said his CEA went down to half of what it was, but he said we cannot rely on the CEA tests completely. The doctor later phoned and wants him to start back on radiation. We feel that maybe another tumor popped up or it has spread more in the bone. The doctor also gave him a script for a pain patch, which we hope can provide some relief.

My Stage 3C colon cancer was diagnosed in March of 2006, and all this time I've been trying to find other Stage 3C survivors who have had a long-term remission, or hopefully permanent healing. It is very encouraging.

During my two years and eight months, my CEA level has been going up and down. The last was 2.8 and I had a PET scan, which was clear.

I've discovered that CEA seems to be a bit of a paradox. My surgeon told me early in my treatment that it was of very little value in the initial diagnosis but it was in some cases a valuable tool to tell if a recurrence had occurred.

My initial CEA at the time of diagnosis was only 2.8. A friend who was diagnosed at the same time with Stage 3c 3 lymphs involved had a CEA reading in the hundreds. One article that I have

read said that a low Initial CEA reading was a
good sign. Since my operation and treatment, my
CEA has sat between 0.7 and 0.9. There are other
factors that will raise CEA. One is smoking and
the other is ulcerative conditions. On one occasion
my CEA rose to 1.2 and an endoscopy found
severe peptic ulcers. My last reading was virtually
undetectable at 0.5.

I had scans done every six months for the first
three years, then yearly for the next two. CEA
was checked every three months for six years,
now once a year. My surgeon does not like too
many scans. Apparently they are the equivalent of
around 600 x-rays and he says that can't be good
for you too often.

My surgeon and oncologist both agree that the first
18 months are a really critical time for recurrence.
I learned that a person could have had some
variations with CEA during chemo and it takes
some time to stabilize.

My husband's CEA has gone up as high as 4.1,
and they no longer seem too worried, as his
scans show no sign of metastases or recurrence.
He is a five-and-a-half-year survivor of Stage
3C rectal cancer and is doing well. His last

colonoscopy showed no sign of recurrence but some inflammation and narrowing of the rectal area, probably caused by the radiotherapy, and maybe this causes his CEA to be higher than we would like. His only problem is some urgency, which prevents us from eating out or traveling. To me this is a very small price to pay when I think back to how ill he was after surgery and treatment. He is now 70 years old and works full time.

CEA can really be a mystery, but I'm glad we have such tests, or "tools," as they call it at the Cancer Center where I go.

My cousin, age 66, had lymphoma, discovered in late winter or early spring of 2007. She finished her treatments last year and is doing great. She also said it will come back in about five years. However, I know a woman who had lymphoma in 1990 and it never came back.

I recently went to my regular doctor and expressed concern over bright red blood in my stool that happened after three times over the past few months. He asked if there was a family history of colon cancer, and I said, "nope, just Crohn's Disease." He said that at that time, because I'm only 25, he wasn't concerned because he thought it was just a tearing in my anal lining, but to call if it happened again more than once. I was so relieved. Of course, not two weeks after this visit it happened again two days in a row, and I also saw bright red blood on my stool in the toilet (not a lot, just a little). I've also noticed that I've been really gassy lately and at one point one day, but only for a minute or two, I had horrible stomach pains, but then they went away. I've been nervous to call my doctor back because I know that's just one more step to something that could possibly be serious. I've also been really stressed out because my fiance and I are getting married next year, so the thought of having to postpone it because of a major illness just makes me so upset. The only other thing I can think of is that I'm not as hungry as I used to be. This change happened over the last year or so. I get full much easier. Also, I had papillary (non-aggressive) thyroid cancer last year, had surgery to remove the whole thing, and have been fine since (and also get regular check-ups). I know I have to call my doctor and probably have a colonoscopy, but I'm just wondering what the odds are of this being colon cancer. Update: I actually made an appointment with my doctor, and they did a rectal and found hemorrhoids, so I'm really relieved. Lots of fiber in my diet from now on!

I had colon rectal cancer six years ago and am okay now, except that my bowel movements are like diarrhea and I really have to run to make it in time. Perhaps if I had more bulk, I would also have more time to get to the bathroom.

I needed to bulk up my bowel movements, so I tried some of the fiber products available over the counter. They helped with diarrhea as well as constipation. But I had to make sure to start slowly and follow the directions, especially making sure to drink lots of water. The ones made from soluble fiber are more gentle than those with bran or psyllium. Some foods that also helped me and are gentle include well-cooked root vegetables, bananas, peanut butter, oatmeal, etc. I had to be careful with the antidiarrhea medications and made it a point to check with my doctor first.

My husband uses Metamucil to bulk up his stools and is not sure if it helps, but he thinks it does somewhat. He recently had to start taking a calcium supplement and that also seems to have slowed him down a bit. The important thing for him is not to cause a blockage, so his maintaining balance is important.

I take Metamucil (1 tablespoon after all 3 meals) and rice for me to bulk up my bowel movements, which in turn makes it easier to make it to the bathroom. There is less leakage. Bananas and peanut butter for breakfast are also a good way to start the day.

I know any information about oral chemo other than that provided by my doctor and searches on the Internet. As for radiation, I learned that they will target the beam directly on my backside since the tumor is very near the sphincter. I don't know if I should take an Imodium before the treatment or wait until I get a problem.

My husband was diagnosed with rectal cancer Stage 3 in March of 2007. He had to take Xeloda and also had to go through the radiation treatments. There were good days and bad days. It was worth it though. My husband had to wear a bag for four months following his surgery, but he did keep in good spirits most of the time. After the reversal, his bowels did have to get used to being used again and he did suffer diarrhea. To this day he is still not what he was before the cancer but

*so far he is cancer free and healthy. I thank God
every day for my husband. He is checked every
three months. It's an emotional road to travel, both
for the patient and the caregiver. Life is different
now, not bad but good. We've learned about
what's important in life after dealing with cancer.
We have a better outlook on life and appreciate a
lot of the things that we took for granted before. I
still wish he never got cancer, but because he did
we appreciate life more. We know he cannot push
himself to do anything but get well.*

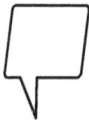

*Before my surgery, I had radiation while taking
Xeloda. The radiation was targeted at my backside
as well because of the location. This process does
cause terrible diarrhea. I took a lot of Imodium.
I began taking it after the diarrhea started and
took it through the whole process. For soreness,
Desitin works the best for me. The radiation wears
you out. But I did drive/go by myself every day.
I wanted to have the power over the process. I
wanted to have control over the cancer!*

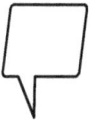

*I had my dry run with radiation. At least now it's
not quite as scary as it was before. I'll get zapped
in three spots. I discovered I was covered with
washable marking pen when I got home. Also I
picked up the Xeloda and Zofran. I also start those*

*soon. I hope that I'm one of those lucky people
who make it through without many side effects.*

SYMPTOMS

The first symptoms of colon cancer are usually vague, like bleeding, weight loss, and fatigue (tiredness). Local (bowel) symptoms are rare until the tumor has grown to a large size. Generally, the nearer the tumor is to the anus, the more bowel symptoms there will be.

Symptoms and signs are divided into local, constitutional and metastatic.

Local symptoms

• Change in bowel habits

  • Change in frequency (constipation and/or diarrhea)

  • Feeling of incomplete defecation (tenesmus) and reduction in diameter of stool, both characteristic of rectal cancer

  • Change in the appearance of stools

    • Bloody stools or rectal bleeding

    • Stools with mucus

    • Black, tar-like stool (melena), more likely related to upper gastrointestinal e.g., stomach or duodenal disease

- Bowel obstruction causing bowel pain, bloating and vomiting of stool-like material

- A tumor in the abdomen, felt by patients or their doctors

- Symptoms related to invasion by the cancer of the bladder causing hematuria (blood in the urine) or pneumaturia (air in the urine), or invasion of the vagina causing maloderous vaginal discharge. These are late events, indicative of a large tumor.

Constitutional (systemic) symptoms

- Unexplained weight loss is a worrying symptom caused by lack of appetite and systemic effects of a malignant growth. However, weight loss is not as much a feature of colorectal cancer as it is of other cancers (e.g., oesophageal carcinoma).

- Anemia, causing dizziness, fatigue and palpitations. Clinically, there will be pallor and blood tests will confirm the low hemoglobin level.

Metastatic symptoms

- Liver metastases, causing:

  - Jaundice

- Pain in the abdomen, more often the upper part of epigastrium or right side of the abdomen

- Liver enlargement, usually felt by a doctor

- Blood clots in the veins and arteries, a paraneoplastic syndrome related to hypercoagulability of the blood (the blood is "thickened")

RISK FACTORS

The lifetime risk of developing colon cancer in the United States is about 7%. Certain factors increase a person's risk of developing the disease.[2] These include:

- **Age.** The risk of developing colorectal cancer increases with age. Most cases occur in the 60s and 70s, while cases before age 50 are uncommon unless a family history of early colon cancer is present.

- **Polyps of the colon,** particularly adenomatous polyps, are a risk factor for colon cancer. The removal of colon polyps at the time of colonoscopy reduces the subsequent risk of colon cancer.

- **History of cancer.** Individuals who have previously been diagnosed and treated for colon cancer are at risk for developing colon cancer in the future. Women who have had cancer of the ovary, uterus, or breast are at higher risk of developing colorectal cancer.

- **Heredity:**

  - Family history of colon cancer, especially in a close relative before the age of 55 or multiple relatives

- Familial adenomatous polyposis (FAP) carries a near 100% risk of developing colorectal cancer by the age of 40 if untreated

- Hereditary nonpolyposis colorectal cancer (HNPCC) or Lynch syndrome

- **Smoking.** Smokers are more likely to die of colorectal cancer than non-smokers. An American Cancer Society study found that "Women who smoked were more than 40% more likely to die from colorectal cancer than women who never had smoked. Male smokers had more than a 30% increase in risk of dying from the disease compared to men who never had smoked."[3]

- **Diet.** Studies show that a diet high in red meat[4] and low in fresh fruit, vegetables, poultry and fish increases the risk of colorectal cancer. In June 2005, a study by the European Prospective Investigation into Cancer and Nutrition suggested that diets high in red and processed meat, as well as those low in fiber, are associated with an increased risk of colorectal cancer. Individuals who frequently eat fish showed a decreased risk.[1] However, other studies have cast doubt on the claim that diets high in fiber decrease the risk of colorectal cancer; rather, low-fiber diet was associated with other risk factors, leading to confounding.[5] The nature of the relationship between dietary fiber and risk of colorectal cancer remains controversial.

- **Physical inactivity.** People who are physically active are at lower risk of developing colorectal cancer.

- **Virus.** Exposure to some viruses (such as particular strains of human papilloma virus) may be associated with colorectal cancer.

- **Primary sclerosing cholangitis** offers a risk independent to ulcerative colitis.

- **Low levels of selenium.**

- **Inflammatory Bowel Disease.**[6][7] About one percent of colorectal cancer patients have a history of chronic ulcerative colitis. The risk of developing colorectal cancer varies inversely with the age of onset of the colitis and directly with the extent of colonic involvement and the duration of active disease. Patients with colorectal Crohn's Disease have a more than average risk of colorectal cancer, but less than that of patients with ulcerative colitis.[8]

- **Environmental Factors.**[6] Industrialized countries are at a relatively increased risk compared to less developed countries or countries that traditionally had high-fiber/low-fat diets. Studies of migrant populations have revealed a role for environmental factors, particularly dietary, in the etiology of colorectal cancers.

- **Exogenous Hormones.** The differences in the time trends in colorectal cancer in males and females could be explained by cohort effects in exposure to some sex-specific risk factor; one possibility that has been suggested is exposure to estrogens.[9] There is, however, little evidence of an influence of endogenous hormones on the risk of colorectal cancer. In contrast, there is evidence that exogenous estrogens such as hormone replacement therapy (HRT), tamoxifen, or oral contraceptives might be associated with colorectal tumors.[10]

- **Alcohol.** Drinking, especially heavily, may be a risk factor.

Alcohol

The WCRF panel report *Food, Nutrition, Physical Activity and the Prevention of Cancer: a Global Perspective* finds the evidence "convincing" that alcoholic drinks increase the risk of colorectal cancer in men.[11]

The NIAAA reports that: "Epidemiologic studies have found a small but consistent dose-dependent association between alcohol consumption and colorectal cancer[12][13] even when controlling for fiber and other dietary factors.[14][15] Despite the large number of studies, however, causality cannot be determined from the available data."[16]

"Heavy alcohol use may also increase the risk of colorectal cancer" (NCI). One study found that "People who drink more than 30 grams of alcohol per day (and especially those who drink more than 45 grams per day) appear to have a slightly higher risk for colorectal cancer."[17][18] Another found that "The consumption of one or more alcoholic beverages a day at baseline was associated with approximately a 70% greater risk of colon cancer."[19][20][21]

One study found that "While there was a more than twofold increased risk of significant colorectal neoplasia in people who drink spirits and beer, people who drank wine had a lower risk. In our sample, people who drank more than eight servings of beer or spirits per week had at least a one in five chance of having significant colorectal neoplasia detected by screening colonoscopy.".[22]

Other research suggests that "to minimize your risk of developing colorectal cancer, it's best to drink in moderation."[16]

On its colorectal cancer page, the National Cancer Institute does not list alcohol as a risk factor[23]; however, on another page it states, "Heavy alcohol use may also increase the risk of colorectal cancer" [24]

Drinking may be a cause of earlier onset of colorectal cancer.[25]

DIAGNOSIS, SCREENING AND MONITORING

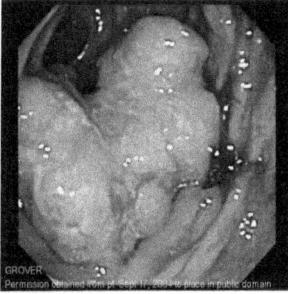

Endoscopic image of colon cancer identified in sigmoid colon on screening colonoscopy in the setting of Crohn's Disease.

Colorectal cancer can take many years to develop and early detection of colorectal cancer greatly improves the chances of a cure. The National Cancer Policy Board of the Institute of Medicine estimated in 2003 that even modest efforts to implement colorectal cancer screening methods would result in a 29 percent drop in cancer deaths in 20 years. Despite this, colorectal cancer screening rates remain low.[26] Therefore, screening for the disease is recommended in individuals who are at increased risk. There are several different tests available for this purpose.

• Digital rectal exam (DRE): The doctor inserts a lubricated, gloved finger into the rectum to feel for abnormal areas. It only detects tumors large enough to be felt in the distal part of the rectum but is useful as an initial screening test.

- Fecal occult blood test (FOBT): a test for blood in the stool. Two types of tests can be used for detecting occult blood in stools i.e. guaiac based (chemical test) and immunochemical. The sensitivity of immunochemical testing is superior to that of chemical testing without an unacceptable reduction in specifity. [27]

- Endoscopy:

  - Sigmoidoscopy: A lighted probe (sigmoidoscope) is inserted into the rectum and lower colon to check for polyps and other abnormalities.

  - Colonoscopy: A lighted probe called a colonoscope is inserted into the rectum and the entire colon to look for polyps and other abnormalities that may be caused by cancer. A colonoscopy has the advantage that if polyps are found during the procedure they can be immediately removed. Tissue can also be taken for biopsy.

In the United States, colonoscopy or FOBT plus sigmoidoscopy are the preferred screening options.

Other screening methods

- Double contrast barium enema (DCBE): First, an overnight preparation is taken to cleanse the colon. An enema containing barium sulfate is administered, then air is insufflated into the colon, distending it. The result is a thin layer of barium over the inner lining of the colon which is visible on X-ray films. A cancer or a precancerous polyp can be detected this way. This technique can miss the (less common) flat polyp.

- Virtual colonoscopy replaces X-ray films in the double contrast barium enema (above) with a special computed tomography scan and requires special workstation software in order for the radiologist to interpret. This technique is approaching colonoscopy in sensitivity for polyps. However, any polyps found must still be removed by standard colonoscopy.

- Standard computed axial tomography is an x-ray method that can be used to determine the degree of spread of cancer, but is not sensitive enough to use for screening. Some cancers are found in CAT scans performed for other reasons.

- Blood tests: Measurement of the patient's blood for elevated levels of certain proteins can give an indication of tumor load. In particular, high levels of carcinoembryonic antigen (CEA) in the blood can indicate metastasis of adenocarcinoma. These tests are frequently false positive or false negative, and are not recommended for screening, it can be useful to assess disease recurrence.

- Genetic counseling and genetic testing for families who may have a hereditary form of colon cancer, such as hereditary nonpolyposis colorectal cancer (HNPCC) or familial adenomatous polyposis (FAP).

- Positron emission tomography (PET) is a 3-dimensional scanning technology where a radioactive sugar is injected into the patient, the sugar collects in tissues with high metabolic activity, and an image is formed by measuring the emission of radiation from the sugar. Because cancer cells often have very high metabolic rate, this can be used to differentiate benign and malignant tumors. PET is not used for screening and does not (yet) have a place in routine workup of colorectal cancer cases.

- Whole-Body PET imaging is the most accurate diagnostic test for detection of recurrent colorectal cancer, and is a cost-effective way to differentiate resectable from non-resectable disease. A PET scan is indicated whenever a major management decision depends upon accurate evaluation of tumour presence and extent.

- Stool DNA testing is an emerging technology in screening for colorectal cancer. Pre-malignant adenomas and cancers shed DNA markers from their cells which are not degraded during the digestive process and remain stable in the stool. Capture, followed by PCR amplifies the DNA to detectable levels for assay. Clinical studies have shown a cancer detection sensitivity of 71%–91%.[28]

PATHOLOGY

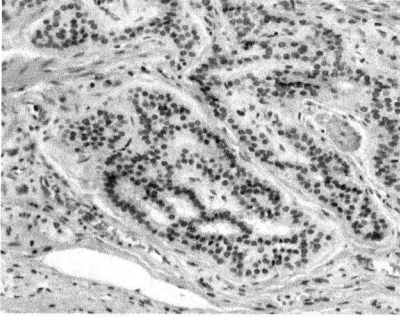

Histopathologic image of colonic carcinoid stained by hematoxylin and eosin.

The pathology of the tumor is usually reported from the analysis of tissue taken from a biopsy or surgery. A pathology report will usually contain a description of cell type and grade. The most common colon cancer cell type is adenocarcinoma which accounts for 95% of cases. Other, rarer types include lymphoma and squamous cell carcinoma.

Cancers on the right side (ascending colon and cecum) tend to be exophytic, that is, the tumour grows outwards from one location in the bowel wall. This very rarely causes obstruction of feces, and presents with symptoms such as anemia. Left-sided tumours tend to be circumferential, and can obstruct the bowel much like a napkin ring.

Histopathology: Adenocarcinoma is a malignant epithelial tumor, originating from glandular epithelium of the colorectal mucosa. It invades the wall, infiltrating the muscularis mucosae, the submucosa and thence the muscularis propria. Tumor cells describe irregular tubular structures, harboring pluristratification, multiple lumens, reduced stroma ("back to back" aspect). Sometimes, tumor cells are discohesive and secrete mucus, which invades the interstitium producing large pools of mucus/colloid (optically "empty" spaces) - *mucinous (colloid)* adenocarcinoma, poorly differentiated. If the mucus remains inside the tumor cell, it pushes the nucleus at the periphery - "signet-ring cell." Depending on glandular architecture, cellular pleomorphism, and mucosecretion of the predominant pattern, adenocarcinoma may present three degrees of differentiation: well, moderately, and poorly differentiated.[29]

STAGING

Colon cancer staging is an estimate of the amount of penetration of a particular cancer. It is performed for diagnostic and research purposes, and to determine the best method of treatment. The systems for staging colorectal cancers largely depend on the extent of local invasion, the degree of lymph node involvement and whether there is distant metastasis.

Definitive staging can only be done after surgery has been performed and pathology reports reviewed. An exception to this principle would be after a colonoscopic polypectomy of a malignant pedunculated polyp with minimal invasion. Preoperative staging of rectal cancers may be done with endoscopic ultrasound. Adjuncts to staging of metastasis include Abdominal Ultrasound, CT, PET Scanning, and other imaging studies.

Dukes system

Dukes classification, first proposed by Dr Cuthbert E. Dukes in 1932, identifies the stages as:[30]

- A - Tumour confined to the intestinal wall

- B - Tumour invading through the intestinal wall

- C - With lymph node(s) involvement (this is further subdivided into C1 lymph node involvement where the apical node is not involved and C2 where the apical lymph node is involved)

- D - With distant metastasis

TNM system

The most common current staging system is the TNM (for tumors/nodes/metastases) system, though many doctors still use the older Dukes system. The TNM system assigns a number[31]:

- T - The degree of invasion of the intestinal wall

  - T0 - no evidence of tumor

  - Tis- cancer in situ (tumor present, but no invasion)

  - T1 - invasion through muscularis mucosa into submucosa

  - T2 - invasion through submucosa into the muscularis propria (i.e., proper muscle of the bowel wall)

  - T3 - invasion through the muscularis propria into subserosa but not to any neighbouring organs or tissues

- T4 - invasion of surrounding structures (e.g. bladder) or with tumour cells on the free external surface of the bowel

- N - the degree of lymphatic node involvement

  - N0 - no lymph nodes involved

  - N1 - one to three nodes involved

  - N2 - four or more nodes involved

- M - the degree of metastasis

  - M0 - no metastasis

  - M1 - metastasis present

AJCC stage groupings

The stage of a cancer is usually quoted as a number I, II, III, IV derived from the TNM value grouped by prognosis; a higher number indicates a more advanced cancer and likely a worse outcome.

- Stage 0

  - Tis, N0, M0

- Stage I

  - T1, N0, M0

  - T2, N0, M0

- Stage IIA

  - T3, N0, M0

- Stage IIB

  - T4, N0, M0

- Stage IIIA

  - T1, N1, M0

  - T2, N1, M0

- Stage IIIB

  - T3, N1, M0

  - T4, N1, M0

- Stage IIIC

  - Any T, N2, M0

- Stage IV

  - Any T, Any N, M1

PATHOGENESIS

Colorectal cancer is a disease originating from the epithelial cells lining the gastrointestinal tract. Hereditary or somatic mutations in specific DNA sequences, among which are included DNA replication or DNA repair genes[32], and also the APC, K-Ras, NOD2 and p53[33] genes, lead to unrestricted cell division. The exact reason why (and whether) a diet high in fiber might prevent colorectal cancer remains uncertain. Chronic inflammation, as in inflammatory bowel disease, may predispose patients to malignancy.

TREATMENT

The treatment depends on the staging of the cancer. When colorectal cancer is caught at early stages (with little spread) it can be curable. However when it is detected at later stages (when distant metastases are present) it is less likely to be curable.

Surgery remains the primary treatment while chemotherapy and/or radiotherapy may be recommended depending on the individual patient's staging and other medical factors.

Surgery

Surgeries can be categorised into curative, palliative, bypass, fecal diversion, or open-and-close.

Curative Surgical treatment can be offered if the tumor is localized.

Very early cancer that develops within a polyp can often be cured by removing the polyp (i.e., polypectomy) at the time of colonoscopy.

In colon cancer, a more advanced tumor typically requires surgical removal of the section of colon containing the tumor with sufficient margins, and radical en-bloc resection of mesentery and lymph nodes to reduce local recurrence (i.e., colectomy).

If possible, the remaining parts of colon are anastomosed together to create a functioning colon. In cases when anastomosis is not possible, a stoma (artificial orifice) is created.

Curative surgery on rectal cancer includes total mesorectal excision (lower anterior resection) or abdominoperineal excision.

In case of multiple metastases, palliative (non curative) resection of the primary tumor is still offered in order to reduce further morbidity caused by tumor bleeding, invasion, and its catabolic effect. Surgical removal of isolated liver metastases is, however, common and may be curative in selected patients; improved chemotherapy has increased the number of patients who are offered surgical removal of isolated liver metastases.

If the tumor invaded into adjacent vital structures which makes excision technically difficult, the surgeons may prefer to bypass the tumor (ileotransverse bypass) or to do a proximal fecal diversion through a stoma.

The worst case would be an open-and-close surgery, when surgeons find the tumor unresectable and the small bowel involved; any more procedures would do more harm than good to the patient. This is uncommon with the advent of laparoscopy and better radiological imaging. Most of these cases formerly subjected to "open and close" procedures are now diagnosed in advance and surgery avoided.

Laparoscopic-assisted colectomy is a minimally-invasive technique that can reduce the size of the incision and may reduce post-operative pain.

As with any surgical procedure, colorectal surgery may result in complications including

• Wound infection, Dehiscence (bursting of wound) or hernia

• Anastomosis breakdown, leading to abscess or fistula formation, and/or peritonitis

• Bleeding with or without hematoma formation

• Adhesions resulting in bowel obstruction (especially small bowel)

• Adjacent organ injury; most commonly to the small intestine, ureters, spleen, or bladder

• Cardiorespiratory complications such as myocardial infarction, pneumonia, arrythmia, pulmonary embolism etc.

My husband had a colonoscopy. He is 44 years old and had it done due to blood in his stool. The doctor told us very good news. He said there was a large precancerous polyp taken out that in another four to five years most likely would have been cancer. He said that we should be grateful that there had been bleeding, because they do not usually bleed, but that it was out now, no worries, have a good day. Then shortly after that, my husband got a call from the doctor saying the biopsy results are in and "after talking with the pathologist I would like you to come in tomorrow to talk about it." Of course, our natural reaction is OH NO!

If a doctor calls one in to discuss results, there could be a list of things he might want to discuss, but I think it is better that the doctor tell a person.

I'm a 48-year old woman who had a colonoscopy because of rectal bleeding (no family history). The doctor removed a large polyp, and the doctor said it looked fine, but it would be biopsied as a matter of course. A week later he called and said the polyp was cancerous after all (he said he knew telling me over the phone wasn't the best, but he said he knew after telling me that it was fine, to make me come in and have that dread for

24 hours would be worse). He explained he had good margins in removing it, but there was no way to know if he got all the cancer, as it looked like it had started spreading into the lining of the colon. When that happens, it can spread into the lymph nodes. I was scheduled for surgery a few weeks later. I was told that most people don't have any symptoms until it's too late. So I was blessed. I walked through the next few weeks in a daze, still feeling like this couldn't possibly be happening. I had the colon resection and for me, the surgery and recovery weren't nearly as bad as I had heard/feared. Long story short, the cancer hadn't spread and the surgeon said I was to "go live my life." What a relief! I decided that it was better to fight the known than to live in fear.

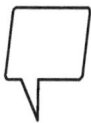

My husband's doctor said that he has cancer after being told he did not. He said that had the cancer been on top of the polyp, no further action was needed, but unfortunately it was at the bottom of the polyp with possible blood vessel involvement so he will need to go in for a colon resection just to make sure it did not spread. He said that it would be very early and that there is a probable 90 percent chance that it did not spread, but they have to check to make sure. We go and talk to a *surgeon and then we will see where we go from there. I know that it will most likely have a good outcome and I trust God completely (at least I am trying), but it's still scary. I am an information junkie so I wish that I had asked for a copy of the pathology report.*

I read about recovery following bowel resection, and I am not sure I found the answer I am looking for. It is now seven weeks since my surgery, and I can do a lot of my normal housework, but I find certain tasks, i.e., those that pull across the body and lifting a little, worrying, so I avoid as much as possible. I am not scrubbing floors or vacuuming at this stage. I am concerned though that I have a sharp stinging pain when I cough or sneeze and tend to bend sideways in the wrong direction. I hope this is to be expected still at this stage. I hesitate to bother my surgeon yet again with another question. I mentioned pain on one side at my re-call appointment and that was normal, but I guess I expected to be a little freer regarding coughing and sneezing at this stage.

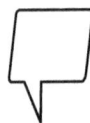

I just had to have an emergency bowel resection. I went in for a dilation and curettage, and my gynecologist ended up lacerating my bowel and I

had to have three inches of it removed. Anyway,
I also have that pain on my right side actually.
It kind of feels like a non-stop annoying pulled
muscle. It goes away after I go to the bathroom. I
asked the nurses in the hospital if it was okay while
I was there, and they ignored me like I was making
it up. As for the coughing/sneezing, I can't even
yell if I wanted to. I am so angry inside and just
want to yell, but I can't. I hope it doesn't last that
long.

I am only one week post-op and still feel horrible.

My post-surgery pain feels like it is linked to using
my bladder. It is now seven weeks and that has
eased up, but with the coughing and sneezing,
I think, there is a back problem, but that is also
easing.

My second round of chemo starts in four days, and
I hope it goes as well as the first lot, but guess I can
expect more side effects as cycles come and go.

I am concerned about a sharp knife-like pain that
always accompanies coughing and sneezing,
but sometimes when moving in certain directions,
while the same movement produces nothing

another time. It also hurts to stand or sit, but at other times all is well. The pain is now on the side of the resection. It is now nearly eight weeks since surgery. I think I should contact my surgeon. I have just come home from a second cycle of chemo and was also wondering if that plays a part in this.

My doctor says post-op pain is normal and part of the healing process. I walked out of his surgery so relieved, and he was right, it eventually went. I still get an occasional odd pain in the area if I have been coughing or sneezing a lot, but it is nothing like the eleven-week pain. There is a term for it and I have always said that the operation and chemotherapy have affected my brain, and just now I cannot think of it. But it is a common occurrence, this pain after surgery, and it is not forever. I think the term is scar tissue.

I had bowel resection and afterward, for 10–12 weeks, I was sure something was wrong with my uterus. I also felt strange pains first on one side and then on the other. I've finally had almost all pains disappear, but I was really worried for quite a while.

I had big operation with removal of a large piece of bowel (due to very bad Diverticular Disease), and I had an ileostomy bag. They had to make an incision at bottom of the scar to allow fluid to drain and I had that dressed for several months. They had to wait for the hole to close up before they could do a reversal, which was not happening. Then all of a sudden I could see the wound filling up, but it did not stop, it kept on going and was getting quite large. It turned out that it was the bowel coming through the wound and was quite large. My surgeon repaired the hernia and also the reversal of the ileostomy. I was in hospital for two weeks, and my stomach looks a mess with the scars. About two weeks later, I noticed the edge of the scar was changing, so I went to the doctor who said it was infected. He put me on two lots of antibiotics. There was no weeping, but one morning I got up and there was fluid trickling out all the time, so my husband took me to the hospital where they admitted me and I went for surgery again the next morning for exploratory and clean-out. They thought there might have been an abscess. They drained off 1.5 litres of fluid, and I still have too small drain wounds, one each side of pubic area. I was in for two weeks again. When I came home, things weren't too bad but then I suddenly started to get this pain. It hit me so suddenly and really hurt and stings and *sometimes lasts a little while. It can come and go many times a day and night. I saw the surgeon and he said that it was probably scar tissue and that I had had a lot done to my stomach and that it would get better in time. That was a week ago, so I don't really know what it is. Sometimes I think it could be something piercing a muscle because when you move, you can get rid of the stinging pain. Sometimes it feels like being stabbed, it is so sudden. Sometimes when you start to walk up stairs, it starts. It has even started when the phone rang one time, so that makes it sound like a nerve thing. I certainly have not strained myself, because my husband does everything for me.*

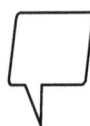

I still have the sharp severe pains in the right quad, and it's been eleven weeks since surgery. I also have a bad time when eating. My gullet hurts and I feel sore in my tummy for about an hour afterward. I wonder when I will feel well again and live life to the full.

Chemotherapy

Chemotherapy is used to reduce the likelihood of metastasis developing, shrink tumor size, or slow tumor growth. Chemotherapy is often applied after surgery (adjuvant), before surgery (neo-adjuvant), or as the primary therapy (palliative). The treatments listed here have been shown in clinical trials to improve survival and/or reduce mortality rate and have been approved for use by the US Food and Drug Administration. In colon cancer, chemotherapy after surgery is usually only given if the cancer has spread to the lymph nodes (Stage III).

- Adjuvant (after surgery) chemotherapy. One regimen involves the combination of infusional 5-fluorouracil, leucovorin, and oxaliplatin (FOLFOX)

  - 5-fluorouracil (5-FU) or Capecitabine (Xeloda)

  - Leucovorin (LV, Folinic Acid)

  - Oxaliplatin (Eloxatin)

- Chemotherapy for metastatic disease. Commonly used first line chemotherapy regimens involve the combination of infusional 5-fluorouracil, leucovorin, and oxaliplatin (FOLFOX) with bevacizumab or infusional 5-fluorouracil, leucovorin, and irinotecan (FOLFIRI) with bevacizumab

  - 5-fluorouracil (5-FU) or Capecitabine

  - UFT or Tegafur-uracil

  - Leucovorin (LV, Folinic Acid)

- Irinotecan (Camptosar) Oxaliplatin (Eloxatin)

- Bevacizumab (Avastin)

- Cetuximab (Erbitux)

- Panitumumab (Vectibix)

- In clinical trials for treated/untreated metastatic disease.[2]

  - Bortezomib (Velcade)

  - Oblimersen (Genasense, G3139)

  - Gefitinib and Erlotinib (Tarceva)

  - Topotecan (Hycamtin)

Radiation therapy

Radiotherapy is not used routinely in colon cancer, as it could lead to radiation enteritis, and it is difficult to target specific portions of the colon. It is more common for radiation to be used in rectal cancer, since the rectum does not move as much as the colon and is thus easier to target. Indications include:

- Colon cancer

  - pain relief and palliation - targeted at metastatic tumor deposits if they compress vital structures and/or cause pain

- Rectal cancer

  - neoadjuvant - given before surgery in patients with tumors that extend outside the rectum or have spread to regional lymph nodes, in order to decrease the risk of recurrence following surgery or to allow for less invasive surgical approaches (such as a low anterior resection instead of an abdomino-perineal resection)

  - adjuvant - where a tumor perforates the rectum or involves regional lymph nodes (AJCC T3 or T4 tumors or Duke's B or C tumors)

  - palliative - to decrease the tumor burden in order to relieve or prevent symptoms

Sometimes chemotherapy agents are used to increase the effectiveness of radiation by sensitizing tumor cells if present.

Immunotherapy

Bacillus Calmette-Guérin (BCG) is being investigated as an adjuvant mixed with autologous tumor cells in immunotherapy for colorectal cancer.[34]

Vaccine

In November 2006, it was announced that a vaccine had been developed and tested with very promising results.[35] The new vaccine, called TroVax, works in a totally different way to existing treatments by harnessing the patient's own immune system to fight the disease. Experts say this suggests that gene therapy vaccines could prove an effective treatment for a whole range of cancers. Oxford BioMedica is a British spin-out from Oxford University specialising in the development of gene-based treatments. Phase III trials are underway for renal cancers and planned for colon cancers.[36]

Treatment of liver metastases

According to the American Cancer Society statistics in 2006,[3] over 20% of patients present with metastatic (Stage IV) colorectal cancer at the time of diagnosis, and up to 25% of this group will have isolated liver metastasis that is potentially resectable. Lesions which undergo curative resection have demonstrated 5-year survival outcomes now exceeding 50%.[37]

Resectability of a liver metastasis is determined using preoperative imaging studies (CT or MRI), intraoperative ultrasound, and by direct palpation and visualization during resection. Lesions confined to the right lobe are amenable to en bloc removal with a right hepatectomy (liver resection) surgery. Smaller lesions of the central or left liver lobe may sometimes be resected in anatomic "segments", while large lesions of left hepatic lobe are resected by a procedure called hepatic trisegmentectomy. Treatment of lesions by smaller, non-anatomic "wedge" resections is associated with higher recurrence rates. Some lesions which are not initially amenable to surgical resection may become candidates if they have significant responses to preoperative chemotherapy or immunotherapy regimens. Lesions which are not amenable to surgical resection for cure can be treated with modalities including radio-frequency ablation (RFA), cryoablation, and chemoembolization.

Patients with colon cancer and metastatic disease to the liver may be treated in either a single surgery or in staged surgeries (with the colon tumor traditionally removed first) depending upon the fitness of the patient for prolonged surgery, the difficulty expected with the procedure with either the colon or liver resection, and the comfort of the surgery performing potentially complex hepatic surgery.

Poor prognostic factors of patients with liver metastasis include:

- Synchronous (diagnosed simultaneously) liver and primary colorectal tumor

- A short time between detecting the primary cancer and subsequent development of liver mets

- Multiple metastatic lesions High blood levels of the tumor marker, carcino-embryonic antigen (CEA), in the patient prior to resection

- Larger size metastatic lesions

Support therapies

Cancer diagnosis very often results in an enormous change in the patient's psychological wellbeing. Various support resources are available from hospitals and other agencies which provide counseling, social service support, cancer support groups, and other services. These services help to mitigate some of the difficulties of integrating a patient's medical complications into other parts of their life.

PROGNOSIS

Survival is directly related to detection and the type of cancer involved. Survival rates for early stage detection is about 5 times that of late stage cancers. CEA level is also directly related to the prognosis of disease, since its level correlates with the bulk of tumor tissue.

FOLLOW-UP

The aims of follow-up are to diagnose in the earliest possible stage any metastasis or tumors that develop later but did not originate from the original cancer (metachronous lesions).

The U.S. National Comprehensive Cancer Network and American Society of Clinical Oncology provide guidelines for the follow-up of colon cancer.[38][39] A medical history and physical examination are recommended every 3 to 6 months for 2 years, then every 6 months for 5 years. Carcinoembryonic antigen blood level measurements follow the same timing, but are only advised for patients with T2 or greater lesions who are candidates for intervention. A CT-scan of the chest, abdomen and pelvis can be considered annually for the first 3 years for patients who are at high risk of recurrence (for example, patients who had poorly differentiated tumors or venous or lymphatic invasion) and are candidates for curative surgery (with the aim to cure). A colonoscopy can be done after 1 year, except if it could not be done during the initial staging because of an obstructing mass, in which case it should be performed after 3 to 6 months. If a villous polyp, polyp >1 centimeter or high grade dysplasia is found, it can be repeated after

3 years, then every 5 years. For other abnormalities, the colonoscopy can be repeated after 1 year.

Routine PET or ultrasound scanning, chest X-rays, complete blood count or liver function tests are not recommended.[38][39] These guidelines are based on recent meta-analyses showing that intensive surveillance and close follow-up can reduce the 5-year mortality rate from 37% to 30%.[40][41][42]

PREVENTION

Most colorectal cancers should be preventable, through increased surveillance, improved lifestyle, and, probably, the use of dietary chemopreventative agents.

Surveillance

Most colorectal cancer arise from adenomatous polyps. These lesions can be detected and removed during colonoscopy. Studies show this procedure would decrease by >80% the risk of cancer death, provided it is started by the age of 50, and repeated every 5 or 10 years.[43]

As per current guidelines under National Comprehensive Cancer Network, in average risk individuals with negative family history of colon cancer and personal history negative for adenomas or Inflammatory Bowel diseases, flexible sigmoidoscopy every 5 years with fecal occult blood testing annually or double contrast barium enema are other options acceptable for screening rather than colonoscopy every 10 years (which is currently the Gold-Standard of care).

Lifestyle & Nutrition

The comparison of colorectal cancer incidence in various countries strongly suggests that sedentarity, overeating (i.e., high caloric intake), and perhaps a diet high in meat (red or processed) could increase the risk of colorectal cancer. In contrast, a healthy body weight, physical fitness, and good nutrition decreases cancer risk in general. Accordingly, lifestyle changes could decrease the risk of colorectal cancer as much as 60–80%.[44]

A high intake of dietary fiber (from eating fruits, vegetables, cereals, and other high fiber food products) has, until recently, been thought to reduce the risk of colorectal cancer and adenoma. In the largest study ever to examine this theory (88,757 subjects tracked over 16 years), it has been found that a fiber rich diet does not reduce the risk of colon cancer.[45] A 2005 meta-analysis study further supports these findings.[46]

The Harvard School of Public Health states: "Health Effects of Eating Fiber: Long heralded as part of a healthy diet, fiber appears to reduce the risk of developing various conditions, including heart disease, diabetes, diverticular disease, and constipation. Despite what many people may think, however, fiber probably has little, if any effect on colon cancer risk." [47]

Chemoprevention

More than 200 agents, including the above cited phytochemicals, and other food components like calcium or folic acid (a B vitamin), and NSAIDs like aspirin, are able to decrease carcinogenesis in pre-clinical development models: Some studies show full inhibition of carcinogen-induced tumours in the colon of rats. Other studies show strong inhibition of spontaneous intestinal polyps in mutated mice (Min mice). Chemoprevention clinical trials in human volunteers have shown smaller prevention, but few intervention studies have been completed today. Calcium, aspirin and celecoxib supplements, given for 3 to 5 years after the removal of a polyp, decreased the recurrence of polyps in volunteers (by 15–40%). The "chemoprevention database" shows the results of all published scientific studies of chemopreventive agents, in people and in animals.[48]

Aspirin chemoprophylaxis

Aspirin should not be taken routinely to prevent colorectal cancer, even in people with a family history of the disease, because the risk of bleeding and kidney failure from high dose aspirin (300mg or more) outweigh the possible benefits.[49]

A clinical practice guideline of the U.S. Preventive Services Task Force (USPSTF) recommended against taking aspirin (grade D recommendation).[50] The Task Force acknowledged that aspirin may reduce the incidence of colorectal cancer, but "concluded that harms outweigh the benefits of aspirin and NSAID use for the prevention of colorectal cancer". A subsequent meta-analysis concluded "300 mg or more of aspirin a day for about 5 years is effective in primary prevention of colorectal cancer in randomised controlled trials, with a latency of about 10 years".[51] However, long-term doses over 81 mg per day may increase bleeding events.[52]

Calcium

A meta-analysis by the Cochrane Collaboration of randomized controlled trials published through 2002 concluded "Although the evidence from two RCTs suggests that calcium supplementation might contribute to a moderate degree to the prevention of colorectal adenomatous polyps, this does not constitute sufficient evidence to recommend the general use of calcium supplements to prevent colorectal cancer."[53] Subsequently, one randomized controlled trial by the Women's Health Initiative (WHI) reported negative results.[54] A second randomized controlled trial reported reduction in all cancers, but had insufficient colorectal cancers for analysis.[55]

> *I knew vitamin D was important so as not to get autoimmune diseases later in life, but I did not know how important a role vitamin D plays in regard to the thyroid. It seems the most doctors are doing is checking TSH and they check T3 and T4 if you are lucky; even fewer doctors do a routine check of the adrenals, and only a few doctors routinely check for the typical malabsorption of various things which people experience with thyroid problems. I received an e-mail from my doctor with some of my latest test results, and my vitamin D is still lower than he would like. When I started out taking supplements, I was below low. I've been on supplements for about a year, and it's been more difficult raising it than I first thought. I never understood why it would be so difficult to absorb vitamin D. My latest results are: 25-OH Vit D 98 nmol/L (48 – 144) Target gt 150. My doctor said that, "Vitamin D3 needs to be improved as it modulates thyroid receptors"; I will ask him what*

this phrase actually means when I see him next week. I did look up vitamin D and found a few things such as:

- Not many endos realize that people with hypothyroid conditions normally lack vitamin D, which leads to some of the bone problems related to hypothyroidism. Vitamin D is poorly absorbed via the small intestine, and this can be Celiac (gluten intolerance) related or that the body may not be activating vitamin D properly. (Celiacs is another autoimmune disease and common with thyroid issues).

- People with Graves also have a tendency to be low in vitamin D.

- Vitamin D and thyroid hormone bind to similar receptors called steroid hormone receptors. A different gene in the vitamin D receptor predisposes people to autoimmune thyroid disease including Graves and Hashimoto #8217s, so it's important for patients with thyroid problems to understand how vitamin D works and to make sure they have sufficient vitamin D.

- When T4 or T3 are low, the body is less able to convert vitamin D into the active hormone and also cannot convert beta-carotene into retinal, the active form of vitamin A. Frequently there is low production of hydrochloric acid which leads to malabsorption of B-12 and iron.

• You can get your vitamin D from the sun (mornings are best), eggs, fish (e.g., salmon and sardines, fish oils, cod liver oil), milk, orange juice, or supplements. You also need normal levels of vitamin D for calcium absorption so that you don't get osteoperosis or other bone-related conditions.

• People with kidney problems cannot convert vitamin D and are placed on something called Calcitriol, as are people who have hypoparathyroidism.

It is cautioned that prior to taking any supplements, not just vitamin D, a person should be tested to see whether he/she is low in that particular vitamin/ mineral. Being too low in something or too high in something can cause the same problems.

Some of the information can get a bit technical. I would advise people to do research of their own regarding their thyroid situation, as there is some amazing information out there that really helps put things into perspective. It makes you realize that it's not just your thyroid and thyroid medication you are dealing with, but there are other organs and other deficiencies to take into account. Don't simply leave it up to your doctor to come up with all the answers, as most of the doctors don't know themselves. That's a bit of an understatement.

I've been reading that many/most people in general are low in vitamin D, especially since sunshine has been demonized in the last thirty years and people spend most of their time indoors now, more than ever (children, too).

There are links between low vitamin D and cancer (most notably breast, prostate, and colon), heart disease, and diabetes.

I've heard that people with dark skin are especially prone to have low vitamin D because the dark pigment in their skin is a natural sunscreen. Their ancestors are from parts of the world that have more direct sunshine and, if they don't live in those areas of the world anymore, that results in lower vitamin D levels.

Everyone should have their vitamin D levels tested and compare their numbers to the optimal ranges.

If vitamin D and sunshine could be patented and marketed to doctors and sold to the public at high prices, it would be advertised on TV and billed *as the new wonder drug. But, that's not the case. People at every age are at risk for low vitamin D and should be tested and supplemented with D3 and/or get a little sunshine!*

MATHEMATICAL MODELING

Colorectal cancer has been the subject of mathematical modeling for many years.[56] For a comprehensive overview of current computational approaches on colorectal cancer see the Integrative Biology web page.

FAMOUS PEOPLE DIAGNOSED WITH COLORECTAL CANCER

- Carolyn Jones, actress and comedienne known for playing Morticia Addams in "The Addams Family". Diagnosed with colon cancer in 1982, died one year later in 1983

- Lynn Faulds Wood, former BBC Watchdog presenter, survived advanced bowel cancer and founded the charities *Beating Bowel Cancer* and *Lynn's Bowel Cancer Campaign*[57]

- Tony Snow died July 12, 2008 at the age of 53[4]

- Ruth Bader Ginsburg

- Tammy Faye Messner died July 20, 2007

- Audrey Hepburn died January 20, 1993[5]

- Lois Maxwell, a Canadian actress, known for originating the role of Miss Moneypenny in the James Bond franchise (which she played in fourteen films), died September 29, 2007

- H. P. Lovecraft, horror writer

- Harold Wilson[6]

- Pope John Paul II[7]

- Ronald Reagan[8]

- Elizabeth Montgomery, American actress (died at age 62; died 8 weeks after being diagnosed with colon cancer; see[9])

- Charles Schulz, creator of Peanuts (died at age 77; died 60 days after being diagnosed with colon cancer)[10]

- Lillian Board, British athlete

- Malcolm Marshall, Legendary West Indian and Hampshire cricketer[11]

- Achille-Claude Debussy, famous French composer[12]

- Bobby Moore, 1966 England World cup winning captain (died at age 51; died 2 years after being diagnosed with colon cancer)[13]

- Babe Didrikson Zaharias, legendary American athlete[14]

- Joel Siegel, movie critic and host of Good Morning America (died at age 64; died 10 years after being diagnosed with colon cancer)

- Eric Turner, second player taken in the 1991 NFL Draft

- Walter Matthau, American actor, had metastatic colon cancer, but died of heart disease on July 1, 2000, aged 79

- Vince Lombardi, legendary coach of the Green Bay Packers, died of metastatic colon cancer

- Rod Roddy, previous announcer for The Price Is Right (died at age 66; died 2 years after being diagnosed with colon cancer)

- George David Low, American aerospace executive and a former NASA astronaut; died 2008

- Corazon Aquino, former president of the Philippines[15]

- Jack Lemmon, American actor, died of colon cancer (and bladder cancer) on 27 June 2001, aged 76

- Sharon Osbourne, British reality TV star and talent show judge, diagnosed with colon cancer in July 2002, aged 49. She is now 55, and is believed to have recovered

- Jay Monahan, husband of news anchor Katie Couric, died of colon cancer in 1998 at the age of 42; Couric became a vocal spokesperson for colon cancer and an increase in screening rates is attributed to publicity generated by her

- Dick Dale legendary surf guitarist whose cancer has recurred as of 2008

REFERENCES

1. "Cancer". World Health Organization (February 2006). Retrieved on 2007-05-24

2. Levin KE, Dozois RR. Department of Surgery, Mayo Clinic, Rochester, Minnesota 55905 *Epidemiology of large bowel cancer.* World J Surg. 1991 Sep-Oct;15(5):562-7. PMID 1949852

3. American Cancer Society *Smoking Linked to Increased Colorectal Cancer Risk - New Study Links Smoking to Increased Colorectal Cancer Risk* 2000-12-06

4. Chao A, Thun MJ, Connell CJ, McCullough ML, Jacobs EJ, Flanders WD, Rodriguez C, Sinha R, Calle EE. *Meat consumption and risk of colorectal cancer.* JAMA 2005;293:172–82. PMID 15644544

5. Park Y, Hunter DJ, Spiegelman D, Bergkvist L, Berrino F *et al.* Dietary fiber intake and risk of colorectal cancer: a pooled analysis of prospective cohort studies. JAMA 2005;294:2849–57. PMID 16352792

6. Gregory L. Brotzman and Russell G. Robertson (2006). "Colorectal Cancer Risk Factors". *Colorectal Cancer.* Retrieved on 2008-01-16

7. Jerome J. DeCosse, MD; George J. Tsioulias, MD; Judish S. Jacobson, MPH (February 1994) (PDF). *Colorectal cancer: detection, treatment, and rehabilitation.* http://caonline.amcancersoc.org/cgi/reprint/44/1/27.pdf. Retrieved on 16 January 2008

8. Hamilton SR. *Colorectal Carcinoma in patients with Crohn's Disease.* Gastroenterology 1985; 89; 398–407

9. DO SANTOS SILVA I.; SWERDLOW A. J. (2007). *Sex differences in time trends of colorectal cancer in England and Wales: the possible effect of female hormonal factors..* http://cat.inist.fr/?aModele=afficheN&cpsidt=2995435

10. Beral V, Banks E, Reeves G, Appleby P. *Use of HRT and the subsequent risk of cancer.* Imperial Cancer Research Fund Cancer Epidemiology Unit, Oxford, UK. 1999;4(3):191–210; discussion 210–5. PMID 10695959

11. WCRF Food, Nutrition, Physical Activity and the Prevention of Cancer: a Global Perspective

12. Longnecker, M.P. Alcohol consumption in relation to risk of cancers of the breast and large bowel. *Alcohol Health & Research World* 16(3)':223–229, 1992

13. Longnecker, M.P.; Orza, M.J.; Adams, M.E.; Vioque, J.; and Chalmers, T.C. A meta-analysis of alcoholic beverage consumption in relation to risk of colorectal cancer *Cancer Causes and Control* 1(1):59–68, 1990

14. Kune, S.; Kune, G.A.; and Watson, L.F. Case-control study of alcoholic beverages as etiological factors: The Melbourne Colorectal Cancer Study *Nutrition and Cancer* 9(1):43–56, 1987

15. Potter, J.D., and McMichael, A.J. Diet and cancer of the colon and rectum: A case-control study *Journal of the National Cancer Institute 76(4):557–569, 1986*

16. National Institute on Alcohol Abuse and Alcoholism Alcohol and Cancer - Alcohol Alert No. 21-1993

17. Alcohol Consumption and the Risk for Colorectal Cancer 20 April 2004

18. Alcohol Intake and Colorectal Cancer: A Pooled Analysis of 8 Cohort Studies

19. Boston University "Alcohol May Increase the Risk of Colon Cancer"

20. Su LJ, Arab L. Alcohol consumption and risk of colon cancer: evidence from the National Health and Nutrition Examination Survey I Epidemiologic Follow-Up Study. *Nutr and Cancer.* 2004;50(2):111–119

21. Cho E, Smith-Warner SA, Ritz J, van den Brandt PA, Colditz GA, Folsom AR, Freudenheim JL, Giovannucci E, Goldbohm RA, Graham S, Holmberg L, Kim DH, Malila N, Miller AB, Pietinen P, Rohan TE, Sellers TA, Speizer FE, Willett WC, Wolk A, Hunter DJ Alcohol intake and colorectal cancer: a pooled analysis of 8 cohort studies *Ann Intern Med* 2004 Apr 20;140(8):603–13

22. Joseph C. Anderson, Zvi Alpern, Gurvinder Sethi, Catherine R. Messina, Carole Martin, Patricia M. Hubbard, Roger Grimson, Peter F. Ells, and Robert D. Shaw Prevalence and Risk of Colorectal Neoplasia in Consumers of Alcohol in a Screening Population *Am J Gastroenterol* Volume 100 Issue 9 Page 2049 Date September 2005

23. Colorectal Cancer: Who's at Risk? (National Institutes of Health: National Cancer Institute)

24. National Cancer Institute (NCI) Cancer Trends Progress Report Alcohol Consumption

25. Brown, Anthony J. Alcohol, tobacco, and male gender up risk of earlier onset colorectal cancer

26. "Implementing Colorectal Cancer Screening. Workshop Summary". The National Academies Press (2008-12-11). Retrieved on 2008-12-19

27. Weitzel JN: Genetic cancer risk assessment. Putting it all together. Cancer 86:2483,1999. PMID 10630174

28. B. Greenwald (2006). "The DNA Stool Test - An Emerging Technology in Colorectal Cancer Screening"

29. Pathology atlas (in Romanian)

30. Dukes CE. The classification of cancer of the rectum. *Journal of Pathological Bacteriology* 1932;35:323

31. Wittekind, Ch; Sobin, L. H. (2002). *TNM classification of malignant tumours*. New York: Wiley-Liss. ISBN 0-471-22288-7

32. Ionov Y, Peinado MA, Malkhosyan S, Shibata D, Perucho M (1993). "Ubiquitous somatic mutations in simple repeated sequences reveal a new mechanism for colonic carcinogenesis". *Nature* **363** (6429): 558–61. 10.1038/363558a0. PMID 8505985

33. Srikumar Chakravarthi, Baba Krishnan, Malathy Madhavan. Apoptosis and expression of p53 in colorectal neoplasms. Indian J Med Res 111,1999;95–102

34. Mosolits S, Nilsson B, Mellstedt H. *Towards therapeutic vaccines for colorectal carcinoma: a review of clinical trials.*, Expert Rev. Vaccines, 2005;4:329–50. PMID 16026248

35. Wheldon, Julie. Vaccine for kidney and bowel cancers 'within three years' *The Daily Mail* 2006-11-13

36. Vaccine Works With Chemotherapy in Colorectal Cancer (Reuters) 2007-08-13

37. Simmonds PC, Primrose JN, Colquitt JL, Garden OJ, Poston GJ, Rees M (April 2006). "Surgical resection of hepatic metastases from colorectal cancer: a systematic review of published studies". *Br. J. Cancer* **94** (7): 982–99. doi:10.1038/sj.bjc.6603033. PMID 16538219

38. NCCN Clinical Practice Guidelines in Oncology - Colon Cancer (version 1, 2008: September 19, 2007)

39. Desch CE, Benson AB 3rd, Somerfield MR, *et al*; American Society of Clinical Oncology (2005). "Colorectal cancer surveillance: 2005 update of an American Society of Clinical Oncology practice guideline" (PDF). *J Clin Oncol* **23** (33): 8512–9. doi:10.1200/JCO.2005.04.0063. PMID 16260687. http://jco.ascopubs. org/cgi/reprint/JCO.2005.04.0063v1.pdf

40. Jeffery M, Hickey BE, Hider PN (2002). "Follow-up strategies for patients treated for non-metastatic colorectal cancer". *Cochrane Database Syst Rev.* doi:10.1002/14651858.CD002200. CD002200. http://mrw.interscience.wiley. com/cochrane/clsysrev/articles/CD002200/frame.html

41. Renehan AG, Egger M, Saunders MP, O'Dwyer ST (2002). "Impact on survival of intensive follow up after curative resection for colorectal cancer: systematic review and meta-analysis of randomised trials". *BMJ* **324** (7341): 831–8. doi:10.1136/bmj.324.7341.813. PMID 11934773. http://www.bmj.com/ cgi/reprint/324/7341/813

42. Figueredo A, Rumble RB, Maroun J, *et al*; Gastrointestinal Cancer Disease Site Group of Cancer Care Ontario's Program in Evidence-based Care. (2003). "Follow-up of patients with curatively resected colorectal cancer: a practice guideline.". *BMC Cancer* **3**: 26. doi:10.1186/1471-2407-3-26

43. Winawer SJ, Zauber AG, Ho MN, O'Brien MJ, Gottlieb LS, Sternberg SS, Waye JD, Schapiro M, Bond JH, Panish JF, Ackroyd F, Shike M, Kurtz RC, Hornsby-Lewis L, Gerdes H, Stewart ET, The National Polyp Study Workgroup. *Prevention of colorectal cancer by colonoscopic polypectomy.* N Engl J Med 1993;329:1977–81. PMID 8247072

44. Cummings, JH; Bingham SA (1998). "Diet and the prevention of cancer". *BMJ*: 1636–40. PMID 9848907. http://bmj.bmjjournals.com/

45. Fuchs, C. S. (1999). "Dietary Fiber and the Risk of Colorectal Cancer and Adenoma in Women". *New England Journal of Medicine* **340** (340): 169–76. doi:10.1056/NEJM199901213400301. PMID 9895396. http://content.nejm.org/cgi/content/full/340/3/169

46. Baron, J. A. (2005). "Dietary Fiber and Colorectal Cancer: An Ongoing Saga". *Journal of the American Medical Association* **294** (294(22)): 2904–2906. doi:10.1001/jama.294.22.2904. PMID 16352792

47. "Health Effects of Eating Fiber"

48. "Colorectal Cancer Prevention: Chemoprevention Database". Retrieved on 2007-08-23

49. Agency for Healthcare Research and Quality (2007-03-05). "Task Force Recommends Against Use of Aspirin and Non-Steroidal Anti-Inflammatory Drugs to Prevent Colorectal Cancer". United States Department of Health & Human Services. Retrieved on 2007-05-07

50. "Routine aspirin or nonsteroidal anti-inflammatory drugs for the primary prevention of colorectal cancer: U.S. Preventive Services Task Force recommendation statement". *Ann. Intern. Med.* **146** (5): 361–4. 2007. pmid=17339621. PMID 17339621

51. Flossmann E, Rothwell PM (2007). "Effect of aspirin on long-term risk of colorectal cancer: consistent evidence from randomised and observational studies". *Lancet* **369** (9573): 1603–13. doi:10.1016/S0140-6736(07)60747-8. PMID 17499602. PMID 17499602

52. Campbell CL, Smyth S, Montalescot G, Steinhubl SR (2007). "Aspirin dose for the prevention of cardiovascular disease: a systematic review". *JAMA* **297** (18): 2018–24. doi:10.1001/jama.297.18.2018. PMID 17488967. PMID 17488967

53. Weingarten MA, Zalmanovici A, Yaphe J (2005). "Dietary calcium supplementation for preventing colorectal cancer and adenomatous polyps". *Cochrane database of systematic reviews (Online)* (3): CD003548. doi:10.1002/14651858.CD003548.pub3. PMID 16034903

54. Wactawski-Wende J, Kotchen JM, Anderson GL, et al (2006). "Calcium plus vitamin D supplementation and the risk of colorectal cancer". *N. Engl. J. Med.* **354** (7): 684–96. doi:10.1056/NEJMoa055222. PMID 16481636

55. Lappe JM, Travers-Gustafson D, Davies KM, Recker RR, Heaney RP (2007). "Vitamin D and calcium supplementation reduces cancer risk: results of a randomized trial". *Am. J. Clin. Nutr.* **85** (6): 1586–91. PMID 17556697. http://www.ajcn.org/cgi/content/full/85/6/1586

56. van Leeuwen I, Byrne H, Jensen O, King J (2006). "Crypt dynamics and colorectal cancer: advances in mathematical modelling.". *Cell Prolif* **39** (3): 157–81. doi:10.1111/j.1365-2184.2006.00378.x. PMID 16671995.Full text

57. Lynn's Bowel Cancer Campaign|http://www.bowelcancer.tv/cgi-bin/page.
pl?page=LynnsStory&accessability=no

GNU FREE DOCUMENTATION LICENSE

0. PREAMBLE

The purpose of this License is to make a manual, textbook, or other functional and useful document "free" in the sense of freedom: to assure everyone the effective freedom to copy and redistribute it, with or without modifying it, either commercially or noncommercially. Secondarily, this License preserves for the author and publisher a way to get credit for their work, while not being considered responsible for modifications made by others.

This License is a kind of "copyleft", which means that derivative works of the document must themselves be free in the same sense. It complements the GNU General Public License, which is a copyleft license designed for free software.

We have designed this License in order to use it for manuals for free software, because free software needs free documentation: a free program should come with manuals providing the same freedoms that the software does. But this License is not limited to software manuals; it can be used for any textual work, regardless of subject matter or whether it is published as a printed book. We recommend this License principally for works whose purpose is instruction or reference.

1. APPLICABILITY AND DEFINITIONS

This License applies to any manual or other work, in any medium, that contains a notice placed by the copyright holder saying it can be distributed under the terms of this License. Such a notice grants a world-wide, royalty-free license, unlimited in duration, to use that work under the conditions stated herein. The "Document", herein, refers to any such manual or work. Any member of the public is a licensee, and is addressed as "you". You accept the license if you copy, modify or distribute the work in a way requiring permission under copyright law.

A "Modified Version" of the Document means any work containing the Document or a portion of it, either copied verbatim, or with modifications and/or translated into another language.

A "Secondary Section" is a named appendix or a front-matter section of the Document that deals exclusively with the relationship of the publishers or authors of the Document to the Document's overall subject (or to related matters) and contains nothing that could fall directly within that overall subject. (Thus, if the Document is in part a textbook of mathematics, a Secondary Section may not explain any mathematics.) The relationship could be a matter of historical connection with the subject or with related matters, or of legal, commercial, philosophical, ethical or political position regarding them.

The "Invariant Sections" are certain Secondary Sections whose titles are designated, as being those of Invariant Sections, in the notice that says that the Document is released under this License. If a section does not fit the above definition of Secondary then it is not allowed to be designated as Invariant. The Document may contain zero Invariant Sections. If the Document does not identify any Invariant Sections then there are none.

The "Cover Texts" are certain short passages of text that are listed, as Front-Cover Texts or Back-Cover Texts, in the notice that says that the Document is released under this License. A Front-Cover Text may be at most 5 words, and a Back-Cover Text may be at most 25 words.

A "Transparent" copy of the Document means a machine-readable copy, represented in a format whose specification is available to the general public, that is suitable for revising the document straightforwardly with generic text editors or (for images composed of pixels) generic paint programs or (for drawings) some widely available drawing editor, and that is suitable for input to text formatters or for automatic translation to a variety of formats suitable for input to text formatters. A copy made in an otherwise Transparent file format whose markup, or absence of markup, has been arranged to thwart or discourage subsequent modification by readers is not Transparent. An image format is not Transparent if used for any substantial amount of text. A copy that is not "Transparent" is called "Opaque".

Examples of suitable formats for Transparent copies include plain ASCII without markup, Texinfo input format, LaTeX input format, SGML or XML using a publicly available DTD, and standard-conforming simple HTML, PostScript or PDF designed for human modification. Examples of transparent image formats include PNG, XCF and JPG. Opaque formats include proprietary formats that can be read and edited only by proprietary word processors, SGML or XML for which the DTD and/or processing tools are not generally available, and the machine-generated HTML, PostScript or PDF produced by some word processors for output purposes only.

The "Title Page" means, for a printed book, the title page itself, plus such following pages as are needed to hold, legibly, the material this License requires to appear in the title page. For works in formats which do not have any title page as such, "Title Page" means the text near the most prominent appearance of the work's title, preceding the beginning of the body of the text.

A section "Entitled XYZ" means a named subunit of the Document whose title either is precisely XYZ or contains XYZ in parentheses following text that translates XYZ in another language. (Here XYZ stands for a specific section name mentioned below, such as "Acknowledgements", "Dedications", "Endorsements", or "History".) To "Preserve the Title" of such a section when you modify the Document means that it remains a section"Entitled XYZ" according to this definition.

The Document may include Warranty Disclaimers next to the notice which states that this License applies to the Document. These Warranty Disclaimers are considered to be included by reference in this License, but only as regards disclaiming warranties: any other implication that these Warranty Disclaimers may have is void and has no effect on the meaning of this License.

2. VERBATIM COPYING

You may copy and distribute the Document in any medium, either commercially or noncommercially, provided that this License, the copyright notices, and the license notice saying this License applies to the Document are reproduced in all copies, and that you add no other conditions whatsoever to those of this License. You may not use technical measures to obstruct or control the reading or further copying of the copies you make or distribute. However, you may accept compensation in exchange for copies. If you distribute a large enough number of copies you must also follow the conditions in section 3.

You may also lend copies, under the same conditions stated above, and you may publicly display copies.

3. COPYING IN QUANTITY

If you publish printed copies (or copies in media that commonly have printed covers) of the Document, numbering more than 100, and the Document's license notice requires Cover Texts, you must enclose the copies in covers that carry, clearly and legibly, all these Cover Texts: Front-Cover Texts on the front cover, and Back-Cover Texts on the back cover. Both covers must also clearly and legibly identify you as the publisher of these copies. The front cover must present the full title with all words of the title equally prominent and visible. You may add other material on the covers in addition. Copying with changes limited to the covers, as long as they preserve the title of the Document and satisfy these conditions, can be treated as verbatim copying in other respects.

If the required texts for either cover are too voluminous to fit legibly, you should put the first ones listed (as many as fit reasonably) on the actual cover, and continue the rest onto adjacent pages.

If you publish or distribute Opaque copies of the Document numbering more than 100, you must either include a machine-readable Transparent copy along with each Opaque copy, or state in or with each Opaque copy a computer-network location from which the general network-using public has access to download using public-standard network protocols a complete Transparent copy of the Document, free of added material. If you use the latter option, you must take reasonably prudent steps, when you begin distribution of Opaque copies in quantity, to ensure that this Transparent copy will remain thus accessible at the stated location until at least one year after the last time you distribute an Opaque copy (directly or through your agents or retailers) of that edition to the public.

It is requested, but not required, that you contact the authors of the Document well before redistributing any large number of copies, to give them a chance to provide you with an updated version of the Document.

4. MODIFICATIONS

You may copy and distribute a Modified Version of the Document under the conditions of sections 2 and 3 above, provided that you release the Modified Version under precisely this License, with the Modified Version filling the role of the Document, thus licensing distribution and modification of the Modified Version to whoever possesses a copy of it. In addition, you must do these things in the Modified Version:

    A. Use in the Title Page (and on the covers, if any) a title distinct from that of the Document, and from those of previous versions (which should, if there were any, be listed in the History section of the Document). You may use the same title as a previous version if the original publisher of that version gives permission.

    B. List on the Title Page, as authors, one or more persons or entities responsible for authorship of the modifications in the Modified Version, together with at least five of the principal authors of the Document (all of its principal authors, if it has fewer than five), unless they release you from this requirement.

C. State on the Title page the name of the publisher of the Modified Version, as the publisher.

D. Preserve all the copyright notices of the Document.

E. Add an appropriate copyright notice for your modifications adjacent to the other copyright notices.

F. Include, immediately after the copyright notices, a license notice giving the public permission to use the Modified Version under the terms of this License, in the form shown in the Addendum below.

G. Preserve in that license notice the full lists of Invariant Sections and required Cover Texts given in the Document's license notice.

H. Include an unaltered copy of this License.

I. Preserve the section Entitled "History", Preserve its Title, and add to it an item stating at least the title, year, new authors, and publisher of the Modified Version as given on the Title Page. If there is no section Entitled "History" in the Document, create one stating the title, year, authors, and publisher of the Document as given on its Title Page, then add an item describing the Modified Version as stated in the previous sentence.

J. Preserve the network location, if any, given in the Document for public access to a Transparent copy of the Document, and likewise the network locations given in the Document for previous versions it was based on. These may be placed in the "History" section. You may omit a network location for a work that was published at least four years before the Document itself, or if the original publisher of the version it refers to gives permission.

K. For any section entitled "Acknowledgements" or "Dedications", Preserve the Title of the section, and preserve in the section all the substance and tone of each of the contributor acknowledgements and/or dedications given therein.

L. Preserve all the Invariant Sections of the Document, unaltered in their text and in their titles. Section numbers or the equivalent are not considered part of the section titles.

M. Delete any section entitled "Endorsements". Such a section may not be included in the Modified Version.

N. Do not retitle any existing section to be entitled "Endorsements" or to conflict in title with any Invariant Section.

O. Preserve any Warranty Disclaimers.

If the Modified Version includes new front-matter sections or appendices that qualify as Secondary Sections and contain no material copied from the Document, you may at your option designate some or all of these sections as Invariant. To do this, add their titles to the list of Invariant Sections in the Modified Version's license notice. These titles must be distinct from any other section titles.

You may add a section entitled "Endorsements", provided it contains nothing but endorsements of your Modified Version by various parties—for example, statements of peer review or that the text has been approved by an organization as the authoritative definition of a standard.

You may add a passage of up to five words as a Front-Cover Text, and a passage of up to 25 words as a Back-Cover Text, to the end of the list of Cover Texts in the Modified Version. Only one passage of Front-Cover Text and one of Back-Cover Text may be added by (or through arrangements made by) any one entity. If the Document already includes a Cover Text for the same cover, previously added by you or by arrangement made by the same entity you are acting on behalf of, you may not add another; but you may replace the old one, on explicit permission from the previous publisher that added the old one.

The author(s) and publisher(s) of the Document do not by this License give permission to use their names for publicity for or to assert or imply endorsement of any Modified Version.

5. COMBINING DOCUMENTS

You may combine the Document with other documents released under this License, under the terms defined in section 4 above for modified versions, provided that you include in the combination all of the Invariant Sections of all of the original documents, unmodified, and list them all as Invariant Sections of your combined work in its license notice, and that you preserve all their Warranty Disclaimers.

The combined work need only contain one copy of this License, and multiple identical Invariant Sections may be replaced with a single copy. If there are multiple Invariant Sections with the same name but different contents, make the title of each such section unique by adding at the end of it, in parentheses, the name of the original author or publisher of that section if known, or else a unique number. Make the same adjustment to the section titles in the list of Invariant Sections in the license notice of the combined work.

In the combination, you must combine any sections entitled "History" in the various original documents, forming one section entitled "History";

likewise combine any sections entitled "Acknowledgements", and any sections entitled "Dedications". You must delete all sections entitled "Endorsements."

6. COLLECTIONS OF DOCUMENTS

You may make a collection consisting of the Document and other documents released under this License, and replace the individual copies of this License in the various documents with a single copy that is included in the collection, provided that you follow the rules of this License for verbatim copying of each of the documents in all other respects.

You may extract a single document from such a collection, and distribute it individually under this License, provided you insert a copy of this License into the extracted document, and follow this License in all other respects regarding verbatim copying of that document.

7. AGGREGATION WITH INDEPENDENT WORKS

A compilation of the Document or its derivatives with other separate and independent documents or works, in or on a volume of a storage or distribution medium, is called an "aggregate" if the copyright resulting from the compilation is not used to limit the legal rights of the compilation's users beyond what the individual works permit. When the Document is included in an aggregate, this License does not apply to the other works in the aggregate which are not themselves derivative works of the Document.

If the Cover Text requirement of section 3 is applicable to these copies of the Document, then if the Document is less than one half of the entire aggregate, the Document's Cover Texts may be placed on covers that bracket the Document within the aggregate, or the electronic equivalent of covers if the Document is in electronic form. Otherwise they must appear on printed covers that bracket the whole aggregate.

8. TRANSLATION

Translation is considered a kind of modification, so you may distribute translations of the Document under the terms of section 4. Replacing Invariant Sections with translations requires special permission from their copyright holders, but you may include translations of some or all Invariant Sections in addition to the original versions of these Invariant Sections. You may include a translation of this License, and all the license notices in the Document, and any Warranty Disclaimers, provided that you also include the original English version of this License and the original versions of those notices and disclaimers. In case of a disagreement between the translation and the original version of this License or a notice or disclaimer, the original version will prevail.

If a section in the Document is entitled "Acknowledgements", "Dedications", or "History", the requirement (section 4) to Preserve its Title (section 1) will typically require changing the actual title.

9. TERMINATION

You may not copy, modify, sublicense, or distribute the Document except as expressly provided for under this License. Any other attempt to copy, modify, sublicense or distribute the Document is void, and will automatically terminate your rights under this License. However, parties who have received copies, or rights, from you under this License will not have their licenses terminated so long as such parties remain in full compliance.

10. FUTURE REVISIONS OF THIS LICENSE

The Free Software Foundation may publish new, revised versions of the GNU Free Documentation License from time to time. Such new versions will be similar in spirit to the present version, but may differ in detail to address new problems or concerns. See http://www.gnu.org/copyleft/.

Each version of the License is given a distinguishing version number. If the Document specifies that a particular numbered version of this License "or any later version" applies to it, you have the option of following the terms and conditions either of that specified version or of any later version that has been published (not as a draft) by the Free Software Foundation. If the Document does not specify a version number of this License, you may choose any version ever published (not as a draft) by the Free Software Foundation.

9 781603 320726